William Acton

The Functions and Disorders of the Reproductive Organs in Childhood, Youth, Adult Age, and Advanced Life

Anatiposi

William Acton

The Functions and Disorders of the Reproductive Organs in Childhood, Youth, Adult Age, and Advanced Life

Reprint of the original, first published in 1875.

1st Edition 2024 | ISBN: 978-3-38283-227-8

Anatiposi Verlag is an imprint of Outlook Verlagsgesellschaft mbH.

Verlag (Publisher): Outlook Verlag GmbH, Zeilweg 44, 60439 Frankfurt, Deutschland
Vertretungsberechtigt (Authorized to represent): E. Roepke, Zeilweg 44, 60439 Frankfurt, Deutschland
Druck (Print): Books on Demand GmbH, In de Tarpen 42, 22848 Norderstedt, Deutschland

THE

FUNCTIONS AND DISORDERS

OF THE

REPRODUCTIVE ORGANS.

THE

FUNCTIONS AND DISORDERS

OF THE

REPRODUCTIVE ORGANS

IN

Childhood, Youth, Adult Age, and Advanced Life

CONSIDERED IN THEIR PHYSIOLOGICAL, SOCIAL, AND
MORAL RELATIONS.

BY WILLIAM ACTON. M.R.C.S.,

LATE SURGEON TO THE ISLINGTON DISPENSARY, AND FORMERLY EXTERNE TO THE VENEREAL HOSPITALS,
PARIS, FELLOW OF THE ROYAL MED. AND CHIR. SOCIETY, ETC., ETC.

FOURTH AMERICAN

FROM THE LAST LONDON EDITION.

PHILADELPHIA:
LINDSAY & BLAKISTON.
1875.

PREFACE

THE FIFTH EDITION.

A FIFTH edition of this book being called for, I have again carefully revised, and here and there recast it. The materials that have accumulated since the last edition was published have been incorporated, and no time or labor has been spared in the endeavor to make the work more worthy of the continued favor the profession has shown it.

I have sought to investigate the subjects treated of, in the calm and philosophic spirit in which all scientific inquiries should be approached, and have striven to keep the text free from any sentiment or expression incompatible with the dignity and the high calling of a medical man.

In conclusion, I would fain indulge the hope that the book may continue to exert, as I trust it has already exerted, some good practical influence upon public health and public morals.

17 QUEEN ANNE STREET, CAVENDISH SQUARE.

TABLE OF CONTENTS.

FIRST PERIOD—CHILDHOOD.

THE FUNCTIONS AND DISORDERS OF THE REPRODUCTIVE ORGANS IN CHILDHOOD.

PART I.

PAGE

NORMAL FUNCTIONS IN CHILDHOOD . . 17

PART II.

DISORDERS IN CHILDHOOD 19

Chapt. I.—Sexual Precocity 19

" II.—Masturbation in Childhood 24

SECOND PERIOD—YOUTH.

THE FUNCTIONS AND DISORDERS OF THE REPRODUCTIVE ORGANS IN YOUTH.

PART I.

NORMAL FUNCTIONS IN YOUTH . . . 47

Chapt. I.—Continence 51

" II.—Celibacy 78

" III.—Early Betrothals. Long Engagements . . 88

PART II.

DISORDERS IN YOUTH 91

Chapt. I.—Incontinence 91
  " II.—Masturbation in the Youth and Adult . . . 99
  " III.—Insanity arising from 109
  " IV.—Phthisis arising from 117
  " V.—Affections of the Heart arising from . . 118

THIRD PERIOD—ADULT AGE.

THE FUNCTIONS AND DISORDERS OF THE REPRODUCTIVE ORGANS IN THE ADULT.

First Division.

GENERAL CONSIDERATIONS ON THE SEXUAL CONDITION OF THE ADULT 120

PART I.

NORMAL FUNCTIONS 121

Chapt. I.—Virility 123
  " II.—Marriage 124
  " III.—Sexual Intercourse in Marriage . . . 132

PART II.

DISORDERS IN THE ADULT . . . 148

Chapt. I.—Marital Excesses 148
  " II.—Impotence 154

PAGE

𝔍. Temporary or False Impotence. . . 154

I. SEXUAL INDIFFERENCE, OR TEMPORARY ABSENCE
OF DESIRE 155
II. SEXUAL INDIFFERENCE AMONG MARRIED MEN . 160
III. WANT OF SEXUAL FEELING IN THE FEMALE, A
CAUSE OF 162
IV. PERVERSION OF SEXUAL FEELING, A CAUSE OF . 167

𝔍𝔍. True Impotence. 168

I. PERMANENT ABSENCE OF DESIRE . . . 168
II. INABILITY TO CONSUMMATE MARRIAGE . . . 170
III. TREATMENT—CANTHARIDES, PHOSPHORUS, ELECTRI-
CITY. MARRIAGE AS A REMEDY . . 184—190

Second Division.

THE SEXUAL ACT, ITS PHYSIOLOGY AND DISORDERS 190

CHAPTER I.—ERECTION . . . 191

PART I.

NORMAL ERECTIONS, OR CONDITIONS ESSENTIAL TO IT 191

PART II.

ABNORMAL ERECTION AND DISORDERS AFFECTING
ERECTION 198

SECT. I.—SLOW ERECTION 198
" II.—ERECTION NOT LASTING LONG ENOUGH 199
" III.—IMPERFECT ERECTION 200
" IV.—IRREGULAR ERECTION 201
" V.—NON-ERECTION 202
" VI.—PRIAPISM, OR PERMANENT ERECTION 203
" VII.—SATYRIASIS 205
" SMALL SIZE OF PENIS 207

INTRODUCTION.

I HAVE in the following pages treated of the *Functions* and *Disorders*, as distinguished from the *Anatomy* and *Pathology*, of the reproductive organs. On the latter topics there are many excellent and exhaustive works, but the former still need much elucidation. Until lately, indeed, many standard surgical writers on the generative[1] system have practically ignored the functional aspect of their subject ; dealing with the whole of the wonderful and complex machinery of which they treat, as if the offices it fulfils, the thousand feelings it affects, the countless social, moral and scientific interests with which it is so intimately connected, were of little or no moment.

A different, and, I trust, healthier feeling has arisen since the first edition of this book was published ; and I think I need not here repeat the apology or defence with which the earlier editions were prefaced.

I have laid under contribution the domains of Natural History and Comparative Anatomy, with the illustrative treasures of the College of Surgeons' Museum, the Veterinary College, and the Zoological Gardens, and have, moreover, availed myself of the experience of practical breeders of stock.

[1] In the following pages the words "generative," "sexual," "reproductive," will be used synonymously ; there are some instances in which distinctions may be made between them, but these are so slight, I need not further allude to them.

I have again followed in this edition the natural division of the subject, and have considered it under the four main periods of—CHILDHOOD—YOUTH—ADULT AGE, and ADVANCED LIFE. Taking each period separately, I have first discussed the normal *Functions* or *Conditions* of the reproductive organs incidental to it. Having fully explained these by the help of the most recent physiological investigations, I have examined the *Disorders* to which each period is most subject. I venture to hope that scarcely a single ailment to which the generative functions are liable has escaped notice. To each it will be found that I have at least indicated the appropriate treatment.

FIRST PERIOD—CHILDHOOD.

THE FUNCTIONS AND DISORDERS OF THE REPRODUCTIVE ORGANS IN CHILDHOOD.

PART I.

NORMAL FUNCTIONS IN CHILDHOOD.

In a state of health sexual impressions should never affect a child's mind or body. All its vital energy should be employed in constructing the growing frame, in storing up external impressions, and in educating the brain to receive them. During a well-regulated childhood, and in the case of ordinary temperaments, there is no temptation to infringe this primary law of nature. The sexes, it is true, in most English homes, are allowed unrestricted companionship. Experience shows, however, that this intimacy is in the main unattended with evil results. In the immense majority of instances, indeed, it is of great benefit. At a very early age the pastimes of the girl and boy diverge. The boy takes to more boisterous amusements, and affects the society of boys older than himself, simply because they make rougher, or, in his opinion, manlier playfellows. The quieter games of girls are despised, and their society is to a considerable extent, deserted. This apparent rudeness, often lamented over by anxious parents, may almost be regarded as a provision of nature against possible danger. At any rate, in healthy subjects, and especially in children brought up in the pure air, and amid the simple amusements

2

of the country, perfect freedom from, and, indeed, total ignorance of any sexual affection is, as it should always be, the rule.   The first and only feeling exhibited between the sexes in the young should be that pure fraternal and sisterly affection, which it is the glory and blessing of our simple English home-life to create and foster with all its softening influences on the after life.

Education, of course, still further separates children, as they grow into boys and girls; and the instinctive and powerful check of natural modesty is an additional safeguard.   Thus it happens that with most healthy and well brought up children no sexual notion or feeling has ever entered their heads, even in the way of speculation.   I believe that such children's curiosity is seldom excited on these subjects except as the result of suggestion by persons older than themselves.

This purity and ignorant innocence in children are not in any way *unnatural.*   It is true that a different rule prevails among many of the lower animals.   For instance, no one can have seen young lambs gambolling together without noticing at what an early age the young rams evince the most definite sexual propensities.   Precocity in them is evidently intuitive, as it cannot depend on the force of example.   This contrast between children and young animals may be explained by the fact that the animal's life is much shorter than that of man, its growth is more rapid, its office in the world is lower and more material, its maturity is sooner reached, and sexual propensities, are therefore naturally exhibited at a much earlier age. In still lower forms of life the sexual period commences yet earlier.   In many species of moths no sooner is the perfect insect produced than it proceeds at once to the exercise of the function of procreation, which completed, its own existence ceases.

Very different should be the case with the human being, who needs all the strength, and all the nutrition he can command for the gradual development and consolidation of his more slowly maturing body and mind.   The completion of the physical frame should precede procreation.   This applies to both sexes alike.

PART II.

DISORDERS IN CHILDHOOD.

IT were well if the child's reproductive organs always remained in a quiescent state till puberty. This is unfortunately not the case.

Amongst the earliest disorders that we notice is sexual precocity.

CHAPT. I.—SEXUAL PRECOCITY.

In many instances, either from hereditary predisposition, bad companionship, or other evil influences, sexual feelings become excited at a very early age, and this is always attended with injurious, often with the most deplorable consequences. Slight signs are sufficient to indicate when a boy has this unfortunate tendency. He shows marked preferences. You will see him single out one girl, and evidently derive an unusual pleasure (for a boy) in her society. His penchant does not take the ordinary form of a boy's good nature, but little attentions that are generally reserved for a later period prove that his feelings is different, and sadly premature. He may be apparently healthy, and fond of playing with other boys; still there are slight but ominous indications of propensities fraught with danger to himself. His play with the girl is different from his play with his brothers. His kindness to her is a little too ardent. He follows her, he does not know why. He fondles her with tenderness painfully suggestive of a vague dawning of passion. No one can find fault with him. He does nothing wrong. Parents and friends are delighted at his gentleness and politeness, and not a little amused at the early flirtation. If they were wise they would rather feel profound anxiety; and he would be an unfaithful or unwise medical friend who did not, if an opportunity occurred, warn them that such a boy, unsuspicious and innocent as he is, ought to be carefully watched, and removed from every influence calculated to foster his abnormal propensities.

The premature development of the sexual inclination is not

alone repugnant to all we associate with the term childhood, but is also fraught with danger to dawning manhood. On the judicious treatment of a case such as has been sketched, it probably depends whether the dangerous propensity shall be so kept in check as to preserve the boy's health and innocence, or whether one more shattered constitution and wounded conscience shall be added to the victims of sexual precocity and careless training. It ought not to be forgotten that in such cases a quasi-sexual power often accompanies these premature sexual inclinations. Few, perhaps, except medical men, know how early in life a mere infant may experience erections. Frequently it may be noticed that a little child, on being taken out of bed in the morning, cannot make water at once. It would be as well if it were recognized by parents and nurses that this often depends upon a more or less complete erection.

PREDISPOSING CAUSES.—What the cause of this early sexual predisposition in a young child may be, it is difficult to lay down with certainty in any given case. My own belief is, that there are sexual predisposing causes. I should specify *hereditary* predisposition as by no means the least common. It cannot be denied that as children soon after birth inherit a peculiar conformation of features or frame from the parent, so they frequently evince, even in the earlier years of childhood, mental characteristics and peculiarities that nothing but hereditary predisposition can account for. I believe that, as in body and mind, so also in the passions, the sins of the father are frequently visited on the children. No man or woman, I am sure, can have habitually indulged their own sexual passions to the exclusion of higher and nobler pleasures and employments, without at least running the risk of finding that a disposition to follow a similar career has been inherited by their offspring. It is in this way only that we can explain the early and apparently almost irresistible propensity in generation after generation indulging in similar habits and feelings. No doubt vicious tendencies are frequently, perhaps most frequently *acquired*. But I firmly believe that moral as well as physical diseases, when acquired, can be transmitted to the progeny.

EXCITING CAUSES.—There are, however, not a few directly exciting causes which can, and do frequently, not only foster this terrible proclivity to early sexual feeling when acquired by inheritance, but even of themselves alone beget it.

We see in some children, at a very early age, an almost ungovernable disposition to touch or handle the sexual organs. This most dangerous habit is not unfrequently, I believe, produced by irritation of the rectum arising from worms. In other instances it arises from some morbid irritability of the bladder. Of the existence of this latter cause another symptom often appears, viz., the constant wetting of the bed at night.

There is, besides, in many persons, as will be mentioned hereafter (p. 77), a morbid sensibility of the external organs, that is excessively troublesome and often painful. This symptom may, I believe, appear very early in life, and, if not removed, lead to consequences that will be aggravated by youthful ignorance and want of self-control. It is to be wished, that all medical men attached to large institutions where young boys are collected, would bear this in mind. However natural the delicacy they feel in investigating such ailments, yet in this, perhaps above all other evils, prevention is better than cure.

Irritation of the glans penis arising from the collection of secretion under the prepuce is another cause which should not be neglected. Since the time that my attention was first called to this subject I have had abundant evidence that the influence of a long prepuce in producing sexual precocity has not been sufficiently noted. In the child the prepuce entirely covers the glans penis, keeping it in that constantly susceptible state that the contact of two folds of mucous membrane induces. We must recollect, moreover, that the child has never been taught to draw back the foreskin, and although the smegma is but sparely, if at all, secreted in early childhood, yet that it may under excitement, make its appearance, and if so ought to be removed, as in the adult, by daily ablution.[1]

[1] Careful ablution of the glans and prepuce every morning will be beneficial for all persons, and if it is neglected, annoyance will be experienced, especially by those who have a long prepuce, from the collection of the secre-

A long and narrow prepuce is, in my opinion, a much more common cause of evil habits than parents or medical men have any idea of. The collection of smegma between the glans and the prepuce is almost certain to produce irritation.

PREVENTIVE TREATMENT.—The first point to be observed will already have suggested itself—cleanliness. Yet I have never heard of any steps being taken by those having the care of youth to induce boys to adopt cleanlier habits in this respect. Children are educated to remove dirt from every other part of their bodies (where it is of less importance in its consequences than it is here), but probably a nurse, parent, schoolmaster, or even doctor, would be somewhat astonished at its being proposed that a boy of twelve should be told (for if not told he will never do it) to draw back the prepuce and thoroughly cleanse the glans penis every day in his bath. In my own experience of the treatment of children, I have found this practice so beneficial, that I never hesitate to recommend it in any cases where there is the least sign of irritation from this or similar causes.

The only objection which can be suggested to recommend thorough cleanliness in early childhood is the supposed risk of directing the boy's attention to manipulations, which may excite sexual desires.

This vague alarm that we must not allude to these sexual matters because forsooth some ill consequences may arise has no longer any influence on me. Daily experience teaches me that much prejudice has too long existed on these questions. I am fully convinced from the acknowledgments of patients that the effects of advice to young men has had no such tendency. Even if the dreaded evil should arise, the same boy who had received such recommendation, supposing the advice was followed by any morbid sensations, would come to the same medical friend and state the consequences, in the full assurance that he would re-

tion round the glans penis; but it should be remembered that this white secretion is natural, and not a symptom of disease. Quacks have frequently so wrought upon the fears of ignorant patients, especially those whose consciences were not clear, as to induce them to think they were laboring under some peculiar affection, whereas a little soap and water would have acted as ceive sympathy and any further advice that might be necessary. I am convinced of the fact that when any such irritation or derangement exists, if the proper steps (of which cleanliness is the most effectual) are not taken to check it, the child will in ignorance handle the organs, and the dangers arising in this way are much greater than those attendant on mere ablution, especially in cold water.

Nothing of course can be more important than carefully to guard against unnecessary manipulation from whatever cause. Children should be early taught not to play with the external organs. Without giving any reason, they may be desired to keep their hands away, which will in most cases be sufficient, if there is no physical exciting cause. The smallest sign, however, of the existence of any such cause should never be neglected. If, for instance, a child wets his bed,—which is generally almost the first indication the parents have of the presence of irritation,— the organs should be examined, and the boy's other habits watched. The irritation is only too likely to determine blood to the part, and the unpleasant symptoms, moreover, show a nervous susceptible temperament, which always requires careful attention.

The cases in which an operation may be required on the prepuce are for the surgeon's decision, and are not within the scope of our present remarks. It has been, indeed, suggested by persons fully competent to form an opinion that the universal performance of circumcision would be of no small benefit. This, however, can be only a speculation. Circumcision is never likely to be introduced amongst us, and there is no doubt that cleanliness will suffice in most cases to remove all ill effects arising from the existence of the prepuce.[1]

---

[1] In a state of nature the foreskin serves as a complete protection to the glans penis; nevertheless to the sensitive, excitable, civilized individual, the prepuce often becomes a source of serious mischief. In warm climates, the collection of the secretions between it and the glans is likely to cause irritation and its consequences; and this danger was perhaps the origin of circumcision. The existence of the foreskin predisposes to many forms of syphilis, and I am fully convinced that the excessive sensibility induced by a narrow foreskin, and the difficulty of withdrawing it, is often the cause of emissions,

Several confessions that have been made to me, induce me to suggest for the consideration of parents and schoolmasters, whether the practice of *climbing* in gymnasia is not open in some degree to objections. The muscles chiefly called into action in climbing are those, the excessive exertion of which tends to excite sexual feelings. Boys have, as I know, sometimes discovered this, for more than one person has told me that, when at school, he had found that he derived pleasure from the exercise, and had repeated it quite in ignorance of the consequences.

I shall not be suspected of undervaluing athletic exercises, but if this particular one has the effect I have described, I should certainly advise its discontinuance.

Those who have the care of children cannot bear this fact too constantly in mind, that the tendency of all irritation or excitement of the generative system, either mental or physical, is to induce the youngest child to stimulate the awakened appetite, and attempt to gratify the immature sexual desires which should have remained dormant for years to come. In a state so artificial as that of our modern civilization, the children of the upper classes are sadly open to this temptation. An enervated sickly refinement, tells directly on the children that are at once its offspring and its victims, begetting precocious desires, too often gratified, and giving rise to the meanest and most debasing of all vices. Of this melancholy and repulsive habit as it appears in, and affects young children, I shall say something here. Its effects in after life will be dealt with hereafter.

CHAPT. II.—MASTURBATION IN CHILDHOOD.

This term, like the word *Chiromania*, can properly be applied, in the case of males, only to emission or ejaculation produced by masturbation, or undue excitement of the sexual desires. It affords an additional surface for the excitement of the reflex action, and aggravates an instinct rather than supplies a want. In the unmarried it additionally excites the sexual desires, which it is our object to repress. Most men require restraint, not excitement, of their sexual instincts. The organs of animals are generally differently formed from those of man, and in them, not unfrequently, the prepuce, besides protecting the delicate glans penis from injury, seems requisite to enable the intromittent organ of the male to be brought into an erect state.

titillation and friction of the virile member with the hand : and in the course of the next few pages such will be the meaning of the term. Use has, however, given it a larger signification. It is now employed to express ejaculation or emission attained by almost any other means than that of the natural excitement arising from sexual intercourse, and in children too young to emit semen, it is liable to produce that nervous spasm which is, in the adult, accompanied by ejaculation.

This degrading practice in a young child may arise in a variety of ways. The most common is of course the bad example of other children. In other cases, vicious or foolish female servants suggest the idea.[1] In such sexually disposed children as have been described, the least hint is sufficient, or indeed they may, without any suggestion from others, invent the habit for themselves. This latter origin, however, is rare in very early life.

As to the frequency of the habit at present among children, or even boys at school, I have been unable to obtain any very trustworthy information. Patients from whom in the confessional of the consulting room, the truth on such subjects is mostly learnt, speak rather of what existed in their day. On the whole, I am disposed to hope that in most *public* schools, the feeling is strongly against these vile practices. Still, every now and then, facts leak out, which show that, even into these establishments, evil influences sometimes find their way, and the destructive habit may take root and become common. In *private* schools, however, which are to a great extent free from the con-

---

[1] I have heard of a vile habit which some foreign nurses have (I hope it is confined to the continent) of quieting children when they cry by tickling the sexual organs. I need hardly point out how very dangerous this is. There seems hardly any limit to the age at which a young child can be initiated into these abominations or to the depth of degradation to which it may fall under such hideous teaching. Books treating of this subject are unfortunately too full of accounts of the habits of such children. Parent Duchâtelet mentions a child, which, from the age of four years, had been in the habit of abusing its powers with boys of ten or twelve, though it had been brought up by a respectable and religious woman. ("Annales d'Hygiène Publique," tome vii, parte 1832, p. 173.

trol of that healthy public opinion that, even among boys, has so salutary an effect, there is too much reason to fear that this scourge of our youth prevails to an alarming extent.

I cannot venture to print the accounts patients have given me of what they have seen or even been drawn into at schools. I would fain hope that such abominations are things of the past, and cannot be now repeated under more perfect supervision, and wider knowledge of what is at least possible.

THE SYMPTOMS which mark the commencement of the practice are too clear for an experienced eye to be deceived. As Lallemand remarks : "However young the children may be, they get thin, pale, and irritable, and their features become haggard. We notice the sunken eye, the long, cadaverous-looking countenance, the downcast look which seems to arise from a consciousness in the boy that his habits are suspected, and, at a later period, from the ascertained fact that his virility is lost. I wish by no means to assert that every boy unable to look another in the face, is or has been a masturbator, but I believe this vice is a very frequent cause of timidity. Habitual masturbators have a dank, moist, cold hand, very characteristic of great vital exhaustion ; their sleep is short, and most complete marasmus comes on ; they may gradually waste away if the evil passion is not got the better of ; nervous symptoms set in, such as spasmodic contraction, or partial or entire convulsive movements, together with epilepsy, eclampsy, and a species of paralysis accompanied with contractions of the limbs." (Vol. i, p. 462.)

Besides the physical symptoms, there are many signs which should warn a parent at once to use all precautionary measures. Lallemand truly remarks—"When a child, who has once shown signs of a great memory and of considerable intelligence, is found to evince a greater difficulty in retaining or comprehending what he is taught, we may be sure that it does not depend upon indisposition, as he states, or idleness, as is generally supposed. Moreover, the progressive derangement in his health, and falling off in his activity, and in his application, depend upon the same cause, only the intellectual functions become enfeebled in the most marked manner." (Vol. iii, p. 165.)

Provided the vicious habit is left off, or has not been long practised, the recuperative power of Nature in the boy soon repairs the mischief, which appears to act principally on the nervous system,[1] for in very young boys no semen is lost. If, however, masturbation is continued, Nature replies to the call of the excitement, and semen, or something analogous, is secreted. Occasionally, the emission gives pleasure, and there is then great danger of the habit becoming confirmed. The boy's health fails, he is troubled with indigestion, his intellectual powers are dimmed, he becomes pale, emaciated, and depressed in spirits; exercise he has no longer any taste for, and he seeks solitude. At a later period the youth cannot so easily minister to his solitary pleasures, and he excites his organs the more, as they flag under the accustomed stimulus. There is a case related by Chopart, of a shepherd boy who was in the habit of passing a piece of twig down the urethra, in order to produce ejaculation, when all other means had failed.

PROGNOSIS.—Evil as the effects are, even in early childhood, the *prognosis* of the ailment, looking on it as an ailment, is not, in children, unfavorable. Lallemand observes:—" In respect to the evil habit in children, it is easy to re-establish the health, if we can prevent the little patient masturbating himself, for at this period the resources of nature are great ;" the French professor does not, however, think that it is so easy to repair the injury inflicted on nutrition during the development of the body ; nevertheless he has seen the consequences disappear readily, and all the functions become re-established ; not so, however, when masturbation occurs after puberty." (Vol. i, p. 468.)

---

[1] Lallemand admits that in children it is not the loss of semen which can produce the usual effects of spermatorrhœa, but that the symptoms must depend upon the influence exercised on the nervous system, or what he terms the *ébranlment nerveux épileptiforme,* the loss of nervous power which follows over-excitement, tickling, or spasmodic affections in young and susceptible children, and which may produce such a perturbation of the nervous system as to occasion even death. He gives an instance of this, which he attributed to the effect produced on the brain by repeated convulsive shocks similar to those which susceptible subjects receive when the soles of the feet are tickled. (See Lallemand, pp. 467–8.)

if proper care be taken to see that boys are well brought up, they will not fall into dirty habits of any kind, much less into so filthy a one as masturbation. And, indeed, it is a good deal to ask of a schoolmaster. He naturally feels that, when he has done all he can in the way of supervision and management to prevent his boys from indulging in evil propensities, the responsibility of warning them against habits which he hopes they have never heard of, and which might be put into their heads if he were to broach the subject at all, is greater than he ought to be called upon to bear. If he were, he says, to discover any boys practising or inciting others to practise the evil habit, they would of course be severely punished or even expelled; but never having discovered such offenders, he does not believe the habit is indulged in at all, and declines to interfere. If recent testimony is to be believed, it is certain that these practices are still (though perhaps less frequently than formerly indulged in). As I have said, it is my deliberate opinion that in many cases it would be true wisdom, and true kindness openly and in plain language to lay before a boy the full extent of his danger, and impress upon him as urgently as possible, the fact that it is a *danger*, and that the consequences of yielding on his part will be most lamentable. I have myself no hesitation as to the advice I should give to parents in such matters. In all cases, I would tell them, the best preventive step to be taken is to watch their children, if not actually to warn them against what it is to be hoped they are ignorant of, and to develop all their muscular powers by strong gymnastic exercises. We must, however, recollect, that it is not the strong athletic boy, fond of healthy exercise, who thus early shows marks of sexual desires, but your puny exotic, whose intellectual education has been fostered at the expense of his physical development.

Little do parents know or think of what they sacrifice in unnaturally forcing the intellectual at the expense of the muscular development. Unfortunately, many of the attempts of modern education tend only to foster intellectual superiority, and children are confined to the schoolroom for hours that, at an early age, had better be passed in the open air.

If such parents would read the biographies of eminent characters who have succeeded in the highest walks of their various professions, they would find that one of the most necessary means of success in life is a strong constitution. If on this be engrafted superior intellectual endowments, accompanied by that energy of character which usually attends the strong, success in after life may be nearly ensured. Youths thus happily gifted are not those whom we see cut off in the prime of life just as they are giving promise of great distinction, and whose parents look back with regret, and ask themselves, with justice, if they have not been partially instrumental in causing these intellectual suicides.

A vigorous healthy boy is not likely to have any tendency to debase himself, and it is a question with many parents if it is wise (on his going to school) to caution him against the vile habit of masturbation and its consequences. My own impression formerly was, that it would be a pity to poison the mind of a high-spirited lad with any cautions about such debasing practices; but my opinion has been altered by the confessions of many who, in ignorance of the results, have, by the example of others, been led to practice masturbation. I believe that in many cases a parent *should* at least hint to his son that he may be very possibly have to witness unclean practices, and conjure him at once manfully to resist and oppose them, pointing out at the same time the consequences to which they tend. There may be the risk of tainting an ingenuous mind by broaching such a subject, and unfolding before it the distressing page in the book of knowledge of good and evil; but when it is needful, a father should in my opinion accept the grave responsibility and ought not to face the greater unknown ill of dismissing his child to the probability of contamination without an attempt to save him. I esteem it false delicacy and a wrong, that a parent should hesitate to warn his boy, when, at the most, he can only anticipate by a few days or weeks the offices of a youthful schoolmaster in vice, as ignorant of consequences as the pupil, and unable to administer the antidote with the poison.

The warning often would not be so unintelligible to a child as is sometimes supposed. Parents are frequently disinclined to acknowledge that their children can have any information on sexual matters. They should bear in mind that, although the father may have abstained from alluding to sexual subjects, yet a mere child, with its keen curiosity, and eyes always on the alert for anything unusual among domestic animals, may already have acquired an astonishing amount of information even about sexual matters—quite sufficient, at any rate, to be very dangerous to him, if not guided and corrected by the admonitions of his parent.

Whatever may be considered the best course for ordinary children, on one point my mind is fully made up. If I saw a child, a few years old, paying attention to female children only, and toying with them, I should watch over his future most anxiously. On the occurrence of any symptoms of debility, paleness, or ill-health, my vigilance would be still greater, particularly if I saw any development of the *idées génésiques*, as Lallemand calls them. In such a case I should have no hesitation in directing the precocious child's attention to the pitfall yawning before him, fully convinced that not only could advice do no harm, but that I should not be teaching such a boy what he ought not to know by calling his attention to sexual subjects. I am of opinion that I should but anticipate the natural curiosity of such peculiarly organized children, who early acquire, from the habit of watching animals, and reading novels left about by their seniors, a smattering of knowledge which excites their feelings, but which teaches them nothing of the ill consequences of the only sexual indulgence they can practice at this early age. To suppose that a parent can keep such a sexually disposed child from a knowledge of much that he had better not be acquainted with, shows a grievous ignorance of the infantile mind. But this mind may be regulated, and the dangerous consequences of the practices may be pointed out.[1]

---

[1] As I was preparing a former edition for the press, a stranger called on me to ask my opinion as to what he should do in the case of a boy of twelve years whom he suspected of evil practices. The boy had fallen away in his studies, had dark patches under his eyes, and was depressed in spirits. In

Although I would not give too much weight to the opinions of sufferers, yet I cannot refrain from introducing the following unsolicited letter from a patient on this duty of parents to their children.

"I fear that you my think me somewhat presuming if I say how entirely I agree with you as to the desirableness, not to say absolute duty, of parents and others duly to caution youths as to their conduct in early life relating to sexual matters. Had my father taken such a course with me, I am fully justified in saying I should not have fallen into an error which I now most deeply deplore. This is all that was wanted, for the strictly moral way in which I have been brought up has prevented me running into any of the excesses of the day. But, of course, I went to a large public school, and there, of course, became acquainted with the practice of masturbation, and almost equally as a matter of course, indulged in the habit, and, without a thought of its baneful consequences, have practised it for years. In fact, I fear you must somewhat doubt this statement, but I assure you it is the literal fact, I pursued the practice from an idea of its necessity, and was fortified in my supposition (so ignorant was I) by the idea that, if omitted, nocturnal emissions supplied the omission of the practice. Besides, I considered it a natural means for allaying the sexual desires, the act relieving me from such desire for some time.

"I see now and regret deeply the great folly of which I have been guilty, but am I wrong in feeling some indignation at not having been put better on my guard by those I considered my instructors? Recently, however (I am now near twenty-two), I happened to discover the disastrous results likely to ensue, and also that nocturnal emissions are symptoms of disease. I, of course, immediately relinquished the habit, never to resume it. I must say, however, that it never had the effect upon me I should have expected from reading your book, inasmuch as I have always appeared and felt strong, healthy, vigorous at school, very fond of play, subsequently well able to perform my daily duties either as regards business or intellectual engagements, and have never been averse to society."

In nearly all young children the practice has only to be left off, and the system will speedily rally. One great advantage in early warning a boy, therefore, is that, as he probably derives little or no pleasure from the act, if he is once put in pos-

such a case I told him I should have no hesitation in quietly talking to the boy without taxing him with any evil practices (which the lad would probably deny). I should tell him that it was well recognized that secret vices are sometimes carried on at school. I should tell him that such practices cannot be continued with impunity, and warn him against them. Steps must, of course, be taken at the same time to improve his general health.

session of the probable consequences, he will very likely abandon the practice. His example and advice may, moreover, deter others, who are not so well informed. So strongly do I feel the propriety of such a course of proceeding in the case of sexually disposed children, that, I would urge parents, if they feel themselves unequal to the responsibility, to transfer the duty to their medical adviser.

I have been so often urged by parents and schoolmasters to draw up a plan which might be of service in teaching them how properly to address children, as well as boys arriving at the age of puberty, that I had determined, in the present edition, to trace out a few notes which might aid parents desirous of following my advice. This has, however, become unnecessary since I read the following advice in a pamphlet lately printed by a clergyman :— "Advantage could, and ought to be taken of the opportunity when a boy says his catechism to explain to him the meaning of some of the terms therein mentioned. When a child is taught 'to keep his body in temperance, soberness, and chastity,' it would not be difficult to explain to him what chastity is, instead of leaving him to find it out, as best he may. He might be given to understand that it does not merely mean that all indecency and foul language must be shunned. The child might be told that he must keep his hands from meddling with his secret parts, except when the necessities of nature require it ; and that any emotions he may experience in those members must not be encouraged, and all thoughts which originate them must be avoided. And when he grows older every boy should be taught that chastity means continence ; that if he would be chaste he must not by any act of his own, or by the indulgence of lascivious imaginations, cause the fruit of his body to be expended. He should be taught that all such expenditure is a drain upon his whole system, and weakens the powers which God has given him to be employed *only* in the married state. He may be sure that 'his sin will find him out,' and if he marries with his powers undermined by unlawful gratification, it will be visited upon his children also.

"If he is old enough to understand the subject, the youth en-
3

combined with gymnastic exercises. If we have reason to suspect any of the other local causes of irritation, such as worms,
stricture, hæmorrhoids, or fissure of the anus, these complaints
must at once be attended to. An account of the proper treatment of these diseases, however, would be out of place here.

Where the fatal habit is actually in existence, there can be no
doubt that those interested in a youth should in the mildest, but
still in a firm way, point out the consequences to which such indulgences lead ; and he should be taught to look upon masturbation as a cowardly, selfish, debasing habit, and one which makes
those who practice it unfit to associate with boys of a proper
spirit. If this feeling can be so far established as to overcome
the tendency, the surgeon can soon remedy the mischief that has
been done by previous excesses. It is, I am convinced, from a
want of attention—in parents, and those who direct the studies
of youth—to the *commencement* of this evil habit, and of a little
seasonable advice and judgment, that many a career begun under
the most favorable auspices, has been thwarted, and many a
boy's mental and bodily powers and growth checked.

Among what may be called the prophylactic remedies for self-
abuse, the *sponge-bath* stands pre-eminent. Its constant use
cannot be taught too early, for it not only conduces more than
any thing to the general health of children, but is within the
reach of almost every one. In the nursery, indeed, and at home,
it is now very generally employed. I see no sufficient reason
why it should be left off when a boy goes to school. Its benefit
is quite as great there as at college or during after life, when,
with modern habits, it is pretty certain to be resumed. In all
public schools, then, its use should, I submit, be enjoined, and I
believe might be carried out with little trouble.

A few words on the method of taking a sponging-bath, so as
to secure the greatest benefit, may be useful. The apparatus
I recommend is a shallow painted zinc bath, such as can be purchased for about eleven shillings. A larger size would be proper
for adults. It should be round, and not of the high-backed
description termed the " hip-bath." With this, a water-can of a
gallon and a half or two gallons capacity, and a honeycomb

Among other preventive measures I should recommend the precaution which is, I believe, now almost universal in schools, that every boy should have a separate bed. This is, as regards the subject we are now treating of, most important, and should be made a *sine. quâ non* in all schools. Evil practices are, I believe, most frequently commenced and practised in bed.

An additional advantage would perhaps be obtained if each boy in a school had not only a separate bed, but a separate compartment in which he might enjoy some sort of privacy.

A conscientious schoolmaster's task, nevertheless, does not end with providing for cleanliness, decency, and exercise among his boys. In spite of all his efforts, masturbation and other vices may spread widely through the school unless a careful supervision be practised. Against these secret evils there is no better safeguard within his reach than a steady endeavour to raise the moral tone of the whole school by means of the upper forms, so that the older boys may of their own accord join in preventing, so far as possible, any ungentlemanly or disgraceful conduct. Without some such auxiliary, the best-intentioned master is almost powerless against the moral infection of such practices.

How diffused secret wickedness may become in schools appears every now and then in scandals so dreadful, that the natural tendency of all concerned is to hush up and forget them as speedily as may be. Indeed it is impossible not to sympathize with the feeling, that to be obliged seriously to doubt as to the manliness, and in a rough way, of the purity of our large schools, would be a great calamity. And in the main this confidence has been no doubt hitherto justified. Still, there are points on which I think all concerned may be a little too confident, not to say remiss. One in particular I wish to mention (I can hardly do more). It seems to be included clearly within the scope of these remarks.

I think a schoolmaster should be alive to the excessive danger of the *platonic attachments* that sometimes become fashionable in a school especially between boys of very different ages. I am not speaking of ordinary boyish friendship, than which there can hardly be a greater blessing, either during boyhood or after life. I would encourage such friendship in every way I could. Growing as it does with the growth of the boys, strengthening with their strength, and cemented by scrapes, fights, sports, sorrows, all increasing their mutual respect and interest, such a manly happy connection strikes its roots so deep as generally to survive most other ties. I am speaking of what schoolmasters cannot be ignorant of—the sentimental fancy taken by an elder boy to a younger, between whom there can be, in the regular course of the school, little natural companionship, and having about it a most unpleasant and dangerous resemblance to passion. I know that such attachments have led to most melancholy results. I have been made aware that some public-school men have declined masterships in their own school because they knew the custom prevailed—would not sanction it—but did not dare to attack it. I have been informed that it has been preached at, not obscurely, from school-pulpits. And I could point to living men, with a wretched burden of recollection from it on their consciences which they would give the world to erase.

I am not suggesting that such modern imitations of ancient platonic attachments are universal, general, or even common in English schools, I only say that they do sometimes exist, and that to the remotest approach to the manners or the morals of the Phædrus the schoolmaster should be sensitively alive.

No doubt it has often struck others as it has myself, how advisable it would be in schools, and, indeed, in all institutions where bodies of boys or young men are collected, to establish, if possible, a kind of public opinion as a rallying point for virtue. There is never any lack of fellowship and countenance for vice; the majority too often favor or support it more or less openly. To make virtue, propriety, self-restraint *fashionable* (so to speak) should be, it appears to me, one of the chief objects at which masters and tutors should aim. With admirable common sense and shrewdness the Rev. Sydney Smith recommends the enlistment of the dread of ridicule, even, on the same side :—" Put a hundred boys," he says, " together, and the fear of being laughed at will always be a strong influencing motive with every individual among them. If a master can turn this principle to his own use, and get boys to laugh at vice, instead of the old plan of laughing at virtue, is he not doing a very new, a very difficult, and a very laudable thing?" It has frequently been done, and by the same means of frank sympathy, thorough earnestness, and spotless rectitude in the instructor, it can be done again. The help which such a tone of feeling would be to a wavering boy is incalculable. Supported by such a " public opinion," a well-disposed boy need not blush when tempted or jeered at by the licentious. Innocence, or even ignorance of vice will no longer be a dishonor or a jest. The better disposed will reprove any immorality, and utterly discountenance all conduct inconsistent with the character of a Christian and a gentleman. No one can have read the life of the late Dr. Arnold without seeing that it was one of the chief objects of his life to establish some such feeling as this among his boys. That he was to a great extent successful those who have had the good fortune to become acquainted with any number of his pupils will be the first to acknowledge.

This manful *meeting* of temptation is not only, in my opinion, a far more courageous, but a far more successful way of disciplining the young to virtue than that sickly, hotbed training, that keeps them more often *ignorant* than *innocent*. Herbert Spencer, in speaking of moral education, has well remarked:— " Remember that the aim of your discipline should be to produce a *self-governing* being, not to produce a being to be *governed by others*. As your children are by and by to be free men, with no one to control their daily conduct, you cannot too much accustom them to self-control while they are still under your eye. Aim, therefore, to diminish the parental government as fast as you can substitute for it in your child's mind that self-government arising from a foresight of results. All transitions are dangerous, and the most dangerous is the transition from the restraint of the family circle to the non-restraint of the world. Hence the policy of cultivating a boy's faculty of self-restraint by continually increasing the degree in which he is left to his self-constraint, and by so bringing him step by step to a state of

and goddesses, omitted to allude to the frightful consequences that illicit love or bestial propensities produce on all those who directly or indirectly indulge their animal propensities."

My ideas on this subject are strongly corroborated by some remarks published by the late Rev. Mr. Robertson, of Brighton, and as they have a practical bearing on the question, I reproduce them here:—"I would far rather that there was much less of censorship of opinion. I know that millions of books, infidel and bad books, swarm out of the press, and yet I would not wish to see them stopped by force, except, of course, such as are shocking to public decency. Great as are the evils of unchecked license in publishing and reading, the evil of permitting any persons to restrict either authoritatively would be immeasurably greater. It is a part of our moral discipline. I would not have that exotic virtue which is kept from the chill blast, hidden from evil, without any permission to be exposed to temptation. That alone is virtue which has good placed before it and evil seeing the evil, chooses the good" (p. 73, "Addresses").

I cannot close this sketch of what the sexual condition of early youth should be—of what dangers and disturbances even in infancy it is liable to—and of the best methods of meeting and guarding against those dangers and disturbances—better than by inserting two letters with which I have been favored on the subject, corroborating, as they strongly do, my own views.

—— Rectory, Feb. 18—.

Dear Mr. Acton,—It is indeed a difficult subject to treat wisely and usefully, but I fully believe you are right in saying that it ought to be faced; and though it is very questionable how far any publication should be placed in the hands of youth, yet good service is done if you supply parents and instructors with such information as shall enable them to speak to individual boys according to their discretion with a confident knowledge of those physical facts on which their admonitions are based.

You are not far wrong, I am afraid, in your facts if I may judge from my experience of three great public schools and several private ones. And if I hesitate to adopt your opinion, it is on the à priori grounds that it is hardly conceivable that the wise and merciful Creator should annex so fearful a penalty to indulgences which the multitude are sure to fall into—indulgences which (unlike the luxuries introduced by art) are supplied—if that is not using too strong a word, for I will not believe they are *suggested*—by nature itself. *A priori* grounds, however, in such a question, are very uncertain ones. I do not know whether the case is the same with the labouring population or with savage nations. If not, we may believe that artificial stimulus brings the upper classes, and civilized societies, under a probation which sifts them justly, and provides for the deterioration and downfall of those who do not stand the test.

I think those judge erroneously who select the public schools as the chief seat of this evil. My own experience is the other way. I used to see it practised shamelessly at a large private school I was at; and, alas! it was known and taught even at a little one, of boys *all below ten years old*, where I was before that. At ——, on the other hand—which I consider far the purest of the three public schools I have been connected with—an open or avowed practice of the vice was sternly repressed by the force of public opinion; and this is more or less the case, I believe, at all of them. The superiority of —— I attribute principally to the influence of the monitorial system, which modern sentimentalism is trying to undermine, and which was far more firmly and effectively at work there than at any other school which has been more especially selected by the assailants as their point of attack. No system, however, can prevent the secret indulgence of the vice, nor the communication of this habit from one boy to another. Parents and tutors may well be assured that, wherever a few boys are gathered together, the evil will become known, however it be regarded by individuals or by the majority; and it follows that such advice as you recommend ought not to be withheld from those who are in danger. Still I dare not urge that the instinctive feeling of the heart should be outraged, or in any way overborne. A hint, a word, addressed to a young boy may often suffice to strengthen the resolutions of purity—a fervent exhortation to chastity and modesty, with a warning that he will be tempted by his fellows to evils which perhaps he is ignorant of; and an affectionate invitation on the parent's part to confidence and confessions, which may in many cases make it necessary, or very advisable, to go much more deeply into the matter.

At any rate, it is very important, as I said at first, that parents and tutors should be fortified with a knowledge far greater than they generally possess on these subjects. I should have found it myself far easier to deal with cases of this sort among my pupils had I felt more secure of my point on physiological as well as religious grounds. And in each individual case, I believe, in that desperate struggle which every one has to maintain in early life who tries to rule his passions by the law of God—every one, that is, who has once let go the reins, and has to gather them up again—it would be the greatest encouragement to know that physical science confirms the dictates of revelation, and to know why and how to look for the aid of nature in resisting an almost resistless propensity.

Believe me, yours very truly,

——.

The second is from a member of one of the universities, who was formerly at a large public school:

——, ——, 18—.

Dear Sir,—In these few lines I will endeavor to state, as clearly as possible, my opinions on the suppressal of the vice which formed the subject of our conversation yesterday evening.

The suppressal of this vice at a school, cannot, I think, be effected by the authority of a master, nor can the efforts of the older boys, though they may forcibly put a stop to any open public practice of the same, compel the others to desist from it. Good, sound, scientific information is what, in my opinion, is required at schools, both public and private.

My first reason for saying this is, that by learning the consequence of this practice, I think a great many will be persuaded, through fear, to discontinue it.

It may be said, however, by some, that the ill effects of it are *known* at schools, but I can affirm that during the five years which I passed at school (both public and private), from the age of nine to fourteen, I never heard that any consequence followed this practice, except the vague one of "weakening."

My second reasoning is this. *Curiosity*, I am certain, from my own experience, and what I have seen at schools, is a great supporter of masturbation. Boys are naturally, from what they hear, curious to obtain some idea of sexual congress. With this intent they resort to the vice, and, with the hope of obtaining more information, they search out all the amorous stories in the writings of classical authors, and in "Lemprière's Dictionary."

This curiosity, of course, causes the mind to dwell constantly on sexual subjects. I think, then, that good information will, by satisfying this curiosity, free the mind to a great extent from sexual thoughts. I will now venture to suggest in what way the necessary information may be communicated to the boys.

It is obvious that if some of the older boys were made acquainted with the subject and not the masters, when the former left the school, there would be no one remaining to impart the information to others.

I should suggest, then, that *all* the masters be provided with such information as is necessary. They might, I think, very well speak to some of the senior boys on the subject, and request them to warn the others of the practice, and exhort them to discontinue it.

The doctor of the place might be considered, perhaps, a fit person to speak to the boys. I think, however, that if he alone were to give his advice, the boys would not perceive that a general interest was taken in the matter, but that it was a subject in which he, as a medical man, was alone concerned; and so probably even *his* advice would not have the influence which it otherwise might. He, of course, by acting in concert with the masters, might do a great deal.

It might, perhaps, be advisable for the masters to lend a medical work such as your own to the senior boys in order that they might see that the ill effects of the practice were not fancies of the masters, but that they were well known by surgeons and other medical men.

Hoping that these suggestions may prove useful both to yourself and the public,   I remain, yours truly,

———.

SECOND PERIOD—YOUTH.

THE FUNCTIONS AND DISORDERS OF THE REPRODUCTIVE ORGANS IN YOUTH.

PART I.

NORMAL FUNCTIONS IN YOUTH.

YOUTH (by which we mean that portion of a man's earthly existence during which he is *growing*—that is, in which he has not yet attained his maximum of mental and physical stature and strength) is, as regards the reproductive functions, to be divided into two periods. The line of demarcation is the occurrence of that series of phenomena which constitute what we call *puberty*. During the first of these two periods, or *childhood*, strictly so termed, the fitting condition is, as we have seen, absolute sexual quiescence.

In the second period or that of youth, which we now purpose to consider, quiescence wakes into all the excitement of the most animated life—a spring season, so to speak, like that so brilliantly sketched by our great poet:

"In the spring a fuller crimson comes upon the robin's breast,
In the spring the wanton lapwing gets himself another crest,
In the spring a livelier iris changes in the burnished dove,
In the spring a young man's fancy lightly turns to thoughts of love."

The dangers as well as the powers and delights of this new energy are increased tenfold. If childhood has its sexual temptations, manhood and womanhood have theirs, infinitely harder to overcome, infinitely more ruinous if yielded to.

Of the real nature of this new condition, of its temptations, of the incalculable advantages of resisting them, and of the means of doing so, it is now my purpose to speak, as plainly and simply as possible.

Dr. Carpenter thus describes the change from childhood to youth.

" The period of youth is distinguished by that advance in the evolution of the generative apparatus in both sexes, and by that acquirement of its power of functional activity, which constitutes the state of PUBERTY. At this epoch a considerable change takes place in the bodily constitution : the sexual organs undergo a much increased development, various parts of the surfaces, especially the chin and the pubes, become covered with hair; the larynx enlarges, and the voice becomes lower in pitch, as well as rougher and more powerful; and new feelings and desires are awakened in the mind."

" To the use of the sexual organs for the continuance of his race MAN is prompted by a powerful instinctive desire, which he shares with the lower animals. This instinct, like the other propensities, is excited by sensations; and these may either originate in the sexual organs themselves or may be excited through the organs of special sense. Thus in man it is most powerfully aroused by impressions conveyed through the sight or touch, but in many other animals the auditory and olfactory organs communicate impressions which have an equal power, and it is not improbable that in certain *morbidly excited states of feeling* the same may be the case with ourselves."—*Carpenter's Physiology*, p. 792.

With this bodily and mental change or development special functions, hitherto quiescent, begin their operations. Of these the most important in the male is the secretion of the impregnating fluid, the semen.

" From the moment," says Lallemand, " that the evolution of the generative organs commences (the testicles act), if the texture is not accidently destroyed, they will continue to secrete up to a very advanced age. It is true that the secretion may be diminished by the absence of all excitement, direct or indirect, by the momentary feebleness of the economy, or by the action of special medicines, but it never entirely ceases from puberty up to old age." (p. 240, vol. ii.)

And now begins the trial which every healthy youth must encounter, and from which he may come out victorious, if he is to be all that he can and ought to be. The child should know nothing of this trial, and ought never to be disturbed with one sexual feeling or thought. But with puberty a very different state of things arises. A new *power* is present to be exercised, a new *want* to be satisfied. It is, I take it, of vital importance that boys and young men should know, not only the *guilt* of an illicit indulgence of their dawning passions, but also the *danger* of straining an immature power, and the solemn truth that the *want* will be an irresistible tyrant only to those who have lent it strength by yielding; that *the only true safety lies in keeping even the thoughts pure*. Nothing, I feel convinced, but a frank statement of the truth will persuade those entering on puberty that these new feelings, power, and delights must not be indulged.

It is very well known to medical men that the healthy secretion of semen has a direct effect upon the whole physical and mental conformation of the man. A series of phenomena attend the natural action of the testicles influencing the whole system; helping, in fact, in no small degree, to form the character itself. A function so important, which does in truth, to a great extent determine, according as it is dealt with, the happiness or misery of a life, is surely one of the last, if not the very last, that should be abused.

But what, too often, are the facts? The youth, finding himself in possession of these sexual feelings and powers, utterly ignorant of their importance or even of their nature, except from the ribald conversation of the worst of his companions, and knowing absolutely nothing of the consequences of giving way to them, fancies—as he, with many compunctions, begins a career of depravity—that he is obeying nature's dictates. Every fresh indulgence helps to forge the chains of habit; and it too often happens in consequence of the morbid depression to which these

4

errors have reduced him, that he fancies that he is more or less
ruined for this world, that he can never be what he might have
been, and that it is only by a struggle as for life or death that
he can hope for any recovery. In too many instances there is
no strength left for any such struggle, and, hopelessly and helplessly, the victim drifts into irremediable ruin, tied and bound in
the chain of a sin with the commencement of which ignorance
had as much to do as vice.

Not that this natural instinct is to be regarded with a Mani-
chean philosophy as in itself bad. Far from it. That it is
natural forbids such a theory. It has its own beneficent purpose: but that purpose is not early and sensual indulgence, but
mature and lawful love. Let us hear what Carpenter eloquently
says on this point:

"The instinct of reproduction, when once aroused, even
though very obscurely felt, acts in man upon his mental faculties
and moral feelings, and thus becomes the source, though almost
unconsciously so to the individual, of the tendency to form that
kind of attachment towards one of the opposite sex which is
known as *love*. This tendency, except in men who have degraded
themselves to the levels of brutes, is not merely an appetite or
emotion, since it is the result of the combined operations of the
reason, the imagination, the moral feelings, and the physical
desire. It is just in this connection of the psychical attachment
with the more corporeal instinct that the difference between the
sexual relations of man and those of the lower animals lies. In
proportion as the human being makes the temporary gratification
of the mere sexual appetite his chief object, and overlooks the
happiness arising from mental and spiritual communion, which
is not only purer but more permanent, and of which a renewal
may be anticipated in another world, does he degrade himself to
a level with the brutes that perish."—*Carpenter, p. 788.*

Shakespeare makes even Iago say—

"If the balance of our lives had not one one scale of reason to poise another of
sensual"—"the blood and baseness of our natures would conduct us to most
preposterous conclusions: but we have reason to cool our raging motions,
our carnal stings, our unbitted lusts."—*Othello.*

"Nuptial love," says Lord Bacon, "maketh mankind, friendly love perfecteth it, but wanton love corrupteth and embaseth it."

Here, then, is our problem. A natural instinct, a great longing, has arisen in a boy's heart, together with the appearance of the powers requisite to gratify it. Everything—the habits of the world, the keen appetite of youth for all that is new—the example of companions—the pride of health and strength—opportunity—all combine to urge him to give the rein to what seems a *natural* propensity. Such indulgence is, indeed, not natural, for man is not a mere animal, and the nobler parts of his nature cry out against the violation of their sanctity. Nay more, such indulgence is *fatal.* It may be repented of. Some of its consequences may be, more or less, recovered from. But from Solomon's time to ours, it is true that it leads to a "house of death."

The boy, however, does not know all this. He has to learn that to his immature frame every sexual indulgence is unmitigated evil. It does not occur to his inexperienced mind and heart that every illicit pleasure is a degredation, to be bitterly regretted hereafter—a link in a chain that does not need many more to be too strong to break.

"Amare et sapere vix Deo conceditur," said the ancients. It is my object, nevertheless, to point out how the two can be combined—how, in spite of all temptations, the boy can be at once loving and wise, and grow into what indeed, I think, is one of the noblest objects in the world in these our days,—a *continent* man.

CHAPT. I.—CONTINENCE.

In the following pages the word "continence" will be used in the sense of voluntary and entire forbearance from indulging in sexual excitement or indulgences in any form.

The abstinence must be *voluntary,* for continence must not be confounded with impotence. An impotent man is continent in a sense, but his continence, not depending on any effort of the will is not what we are now speaking of.

Nor is the continence which I advise, and would encourage by every means in my power, mere absence of desire arising from ignorance. That, as I have already said, p. 41, I consider a dangerous condition. True continence is complete control over the passions, exercised by one who has felt their power, and who, were it not for his steady will, not only could, but would indulge them.

Again, continence must be *entire*. The fact of the indulgence being lawful or unlawful, does not affect the question of continence. In this respect our definition differs from those in most dictionaries.[1]

This definition, of course, excludes the masturbator from the category of continent men, even though he may never have had connection with a female. It can only be in a loose and inaccurate sense that an Onanist can be called continent. He is not really so. Continence consists not only in abstaining from sexual congress, but in controlling all sexual excitement. If a young man indulge in masturbation it is easy enough, as will be presently shown, for him to abstain from fornication. In fact, the one is generally incompatible with the other.

We may confidently assert that no man is entitled to the character of being continent or chaste who by any unnatural means causes expulsion of semen. On the other hand, the occasional occurrence of nocturnal emissions or wet dreams is quite compatible with and, indeed, is to be expected as a consequence of continence, whether temporary or permanent. It is in this way that nature relieves herself. Any voluntary imitation or excitement of this process is, in every sense of the word, incontinence. I would exclude from the category of continent men those (and they are more numerous than may be generally supposed) who actually forbear from sexual intercourse, but put no restraint

---

[1] The following are one or two of the definitions of the word " continence" in standard works :

" Abstinence from, or moderation in, the pleasures of physical love."—*R. Dunglison, M.D.*

" The abstaining from unlawful pleasures."—*Bailey.*

" Forbearance of lawful pleasure."—*Ash.*

upon impure thoughts or the indulgence of sexual excitement, provided intercourse does not follow. This is only physical continence: it is incomplete without mental continence also.

Such men as these, supposing the sexual excitement is followed by nocturnal emissions, as it often is, and this with great detriment to the nervous system, must not be ranked with the continents; to all intents and purposes they are ONANISTS. The subject will be further discussed in the chapter on ungratified sexual excitement.

THE ADVANTAGES OF CONTINENCE.—If a healthy, well-disposed boy has been properly educated, by the time he arrives at the age of fourteen or sixteen he possesses a frame approaching its full vigor. His conscience is unburdened, his intellect clear, his address frank and candid, his memory good, his spirits are buoyant, his complexion is bright. Every function of the body is well performed, and no fatigue is felt after moderate exertion. The youth evinces that elasticity of body and that happy control of himself and his feelings which are indicative of the robust health and absence of care which should accompany youth. His whole time is given up to his studies and amusements, and as he feels his stature increase and his intellect enlarge, he gladly prepares for his coming struggle with the world.

The advantages of chastity have been well put by Professor Newman in a pamphlet he has published on the "Relation of Physiology to Sexual Morals." Although, as I shall have occasion to remark, I entirely disagree with him on many of the principles advanced in other parts of his book, I think he has done good service in making the following observations, which I generally coincide in, and which I prefer to quote rather than attempt to epitomize:

"Moralists have at all times regarded strict temperance in food, and abstinence from strong drinks, to be of cardinal value in the maintenance of young men's purity. But whatever our care to be temperate, whatever our activity of body, it is not possible always to keep the exact balance between supply and bodily need. Every organ is liable occasionally to be overcharged, and, *in every youthful or vigorous nature*, has power to

induced by any voluntary act of the person, and without any previous mental inflammation : next, that it occasionally comes upon married men, when circumstances put them for long together in the position of the unmarried; moreover, even when they become elderly, it does not wholly forsake them under such circumstances. My belief is that it is a sign of vigor. At any rate I assert most positively that it is an utter mistake to suppose that it necessarily weakens or depresses, or entails any disagreeable after-results whatever. I have never so much as once in my life had reason to think so. I have even believed that it adds to the spring of the body, and to the pride of manhood in youths. Of course there is an amount of starvation (at least I assume there is), which would supersede it; but to overdo the starvation even a little, may be an error on the wrong side.—And again, there is probably an amount of athletic practice which will take up all the supplies of full nutriment in the intensifying of muscle or of vital force, and leave no sexual superfluity. But labor so severe is stupefying to the brain and very unfavorable to high mental action. Plato is not alone in regarding athletes as unintellectual. Aristotle deprecates their system of 'overfeeding and overworking.' And after all, you will not succeed in exactly keeping the balance, whether you try by starvation or by toil; and the over careful effort will but produce either a valetudinarian, or else a religious ascetic, who is in terrible alarm lest Nature inflict upon him a momentary animal pleasure. A state of anxiety and tremor is not mentally wholesome. We must take things as they come, observing broad rules of moderation as wisely as we can, but without nervous alarm about details. The advantages of vegetarian food I have learned only late in life. I now know that I might have been wiser in my diet. With better knowledge I should have done far better as to the *quality* of food; but I do not easily believe that a more scrupulous dread of satisfying my appetite lest it cause some small sexual superfluity would have conduced either to mental or to bodily health, at any time of my life, unmarried or married."—Page 26.

If, then, the above are the advantages of continence, let us

ordinary effort; and every year of voluntary chastity renders the task easier by the mere force of habit.

Yet it can hardly be denied that a very considerable number, even of the more or less pure, do suffer, at least temporarily, no little distress.

Lallemand has given a vivid sketch of this sexual uneasiness, which the early recollections of many of my readers may verify. "There is a constant state of orgasm and erotic preoccupation, accompanied with agitation, disquiet, and *malaise*, an indefinable derangement of all the functions. This state of distress is seen particularly in young men who have arrived at puberty, and whose innocence has been preserved from any unfortunate initiation. Their disposition becomes soured, impatient and sad. They fall into a state of melancholy or misanthropy, sometimes become disgusted with life, and are disposed to shed tears without any cause. They seek solitude in order to dream about the great mystery which absorbs them; about those great unknown passions which cause their blood to boil. They are at the same time restless and apathetic, agitated and drowsy. Their head is in a state of fermentation, and nevertheless weighed down by a sort of habitual headache. A spontaneous emission or escape, which causes this state of plethora to cease, is a true and salutary crisis which for the moment re-establishes the equilibrium of the economy." (Vol. II, p. 324.)

I have quoted this passage as containing a brilliant, though, perhaps rather exaggerated sketch of a state of mind and body that is very common, and is the chief difficulty in the way of a youth's remaining chaste. I am, however, far from endorsing the author's remark, that this distress affects those particularly "whose innocence has been preserved from any unfortunate initiations." On the contrary, it is my experience that these are just the persons who are, generally speaking, too happy and healthy to be troubled with these importunate weaknesses. The *semi-continent*, the men who indeed see the better course, and approve of it, but follow the worse—the men who, without any of the recklessness of the hardened sensualist, or any of the strength of the conscientiously pure man, endure at once the sufferings of self-denial and the remorse of self-indulgence—these are the men of whom Lallemand's words are a living description.

The facts which show the truth of this are innumerable, and apply to the youth, of whom I am now more particularly speaking, as much as to the adult.   It is a matter of everyday experience to hear patients complain that a state of continence after a certain time produces a most irritable condition of the nervous system, so that the individual is unable to settle his mind to anything:—study becomes impossible; the student cannot sit still; sedentary occupations are unbearable, and sexual ideas intrude perpetually on the patient's thoughts.   When this complaint is made, there is little doubt what confession is coming next—a confession that at once explains the symptoms.   Of course in such cases the self-prescribed remedy has been most effective, and sexual intercourse has enabled the student at once to recommence his labors, the poet his verses, and the faded imagination of the painter to resume its fervor and its brilliancy; while the writer who for days has not been able to construct two phrases that he considered readable, has found himself, after relief of the seminal vessels, in a condition to dictate his best performances. Of course with such persons continence is sure to induce this state of irritability.   Still, no such symptoms, however feelingly described, should ever induce a medical man even to seem to sanction his patient's continuing the fatal remedy, which is only perpetuating the disease.

In all solemn earnestness I protest against such false treatment.   It is better for a youth to live a continent life.   The *strictly* continent suffer little or none of this irritability ; but the incontinent, as soon as seminal plethora occurs, are sure to be troubled in one or other of the ways above spoken of : while the remedy of indulgence, if effective, requires repetition as often as the inconvenience returns.   If instead of gratifying his inclinations the young patient consults a medical man, he should be told, and the result would soon prove the correctness of the advice given, that attention to diet, aperient medicine (if necessary), gymnastic exercises, and self-control, will most effectually relieve the symptoms; and precautions mentioned in the chapter on Nocturnal Emissions will prevent a repetition of the seminal plethora.

The truth is, that most people, and especially the young, are only too glad to find an excuse for *indulging* their animal propensities, instead of endeavoring to regulate or control them. I have not a doubt that this sexual suffering is often much exaggerated, if not invented, for this purpose. Even where it really exists (and I am free to confess that in certain individuals continence of the sexual feelings is very difficult), one of the last remedies the patient would entertain the idea of, would be, that first recommended by a conscientious professional man, viz., attention to diet—exercise—and, in fact, regimen. That there should be more testimony in favor of the remedy considered agreeable than that of involving constraint or inconvenience, is easily explicable on the supposition that the witnesses have not had experience of both systems.

If any one wished to undergo the acutest sexual suffering, he could adopt no more certain method than to be incontinent, with the intention of becoming continent again, when he had "sown his wild oats." The agony of breaking off a habit which so rapidly entwines itself with every fibre of the human frame is such that it would not be too much to say to any young man commencing a career of vice—"You are going a road on which you will *never* turn back. However much you may wish it the struggle will be too much for you. You had better stop now. It is your last chance."

There is a terrible significance in the Wise Man's words, "*None* that go to her return again, neither take they hold on the paths of life."

How much more severe, occasional incontinence makes the necessary struggle to remain continent at all, appears from the sexual distress which widowers, or those married men to whom access to their wives is forbidden, suffer.

That this is not only the result of my experience, I will quote the statement of my friend Dr. ——, who is constantly attending for serious diseases of the womb the wives of clergymen, as well as of Dissenting ministers, in whose cases, for months together, marital intercourse is necessarily forbidden. He tells me that he has often been surprised at the amount of sexual suffering—the result of their compulsory celibacy—endured by the husbands of some of his patients—men in every other relation of life most determined and energetic. Indeed it is not wonderful that it should be so, if we consider the position of such men, who for years may have indulged with moderation, the sex-passion as we have described it, untrained to mortification in the shape of food or exercise, or marital intercourse, the secretion of perfect semen going on in obedience to the healthy course of a married man's existence. Conceive them reined up suddenly, as it were, and bidden to do battle with their instincts. Religion and morality prevent them, more than others, from having sexual intercourse with strange women; intense interest on the subject of the sex-passion in general, as well as misapprehension of the effects of the disease of the generative organs, only aggravates their suffering; conceive all this, and it is not difficult to believe that affections of the brain may supervene.

These remarks are in no way intended as any excuse or palliation for incontinence, but as warnings to the young. These, it must be remembered, are the complaints of *incontinent* men, and I mention them here to show how much easier it is even in adult life to abstain altogether than it is to control the feelings, when they have been once excited and indulged. The real remedy for sexual distress is resolute continence and the use of all the hygienic aids in our power—not the quack receipt of indulgence with the futile intention of curing the incontinence afterwards.

The admitted fact that continence, even at the very beginning of manhood, is frequently productive of distress, is often a struggle hard to be borne,—still harder to be completely victorious in,—is not to be at all regarded as an argument that it is an *evil*. A thoughtful writer has on this subject some admirable remarks :—" Providence has seen it necessary to make very ample provision for the preservation and utmost possible extension of all species. The aim seems to diffuse existence as widely as possible, to fill up every vacant piece of space with some sentiment being, to be a vehicle of enjoyment. Hence this passion is conferred in great force. But the relation between the number of beings and the means of supporting them is only on the footing of a general law. There may be occasional discrepancy between the laws operating for the multiplication of individuals and the laws operating to supply them with the means of subsistence, and evils will be endured in consequence, even in our own highly favored species; but against all these evils and against those numberless vexations which have arisen in all ages from the attachment of the sexes, place the vast amount of happiness which is derived from this source—the centre of the whole circle of the domestic affections, the sweetening principle of life, the prompter of all our most generous feelings and even of our most virtuous resolves and exertions—and every ill that can be traced to it is but as dust in the balance. And here also we must be on our guard against judging from what we see in the world at a particular era. As reason and the higher sentiments of man's nature increase in force, this passion is put under better regulation, so as to lessen many of the evils connected with it. The civilized man is more able to give it due control; his attachments are less the result of impulse; he studies more the weal of his partner and offspring. There are even some of the resentful feelings connected in early society with love, such as hatred of successful rivalry, and jealousy, which almost disappear in an advanced state of civilization. The evil springing, in our own species at least, from this passion may, therefore, be an exception mainly peculiar to a particular term of the world's progress, and which may be expected to decrease greatly in amount."[1]

In addition to the foregoing considerations, I would venture to suggest one that should not be forgotten. Granted that continence is a *trial*, a sore trial, a bitter trial, if you will—what, I would ask, is the use or object of a trial but to *try*, to test, to elicit, strengthen and brace, whatever of sterling, whatever of valuable, there is in the thing tried? To yield at once—is this the right way to meet a trial? To lay down one's arms at the first threatening of conflict—is this a *creditable* escape from trial,

---

[1] "Vestiges of Creation," tenth edition, p. 310.

to say no more? Nay, is it *safe*, when the trial is imposed by the highest possible authority?

"The first use," says the late Rev. F. Robertson, "a man makes of every power or talent given to him is a bad use. The first time a man ever uses a flail it is to the injury of his own head and of those who stand around him. The first time a child has a sharp-edged tool in his hand he cuts his finger. But this is no reason why he should not be ever taught to use a knife. The first use a man makes of his affections is to sensualize his spirit. Yet he cannot be ennobled except through those very affections. The first time a kingdom is put in possession of liberty the result is anarchy. The first time a man is put in possession of intellectual knowledge he is conscious of the approaches of sceptical feeling. But that is no proof that liberty is bad or that instruction should not be given. It is a law of our humanity that man must know both good and evil; he must know good *through* evil. There never was a principle but what triumphed through much evil; no man ever progressed to greatness and goodness but through great mistakes."[1]

The argument in favor of the great mental, moral, and physical advantage of early continence does not want for high secular authority and countenance, as the recollection of the least learned reader will suggest in a moment. Let us be content here with the wise Greek,[2] who, to the question when men should love, answered, "A young man, not yet; an old man, not at all;" and with the still wiser Englishman,[3] who thus writes:—"You may observe that amongst all the great and worthy persons (whereof the memory remaineth, either ancient or recent) there is not one that hath been transported to the mad degree of love —which shows that great spirits and great business do keep out this weak passion. . . . . . By how much the more ought men to beware of this passion, which loseth not only other things, but itself. As for the other losses, the poet's relation doth well figure them:—'*That he that preferred Helena quitted the gifts of Juno and Pallas ;*' for whosoever esteemeth too much of amor-

---

[1] Robertson's "Discourses," pages 87, 88.
[2] Thales.   [3] Lord Bacon.

ous affection, quitteth both riches and wisdom. . . . . They do best, who, if they cannot but admit love, yet make it keep quarter."

AIDS TO CONTINENCE.—Every wise man must feel that no help is to be despised in any part of the life-battle all have to fight. And in that struggle for purity, which is, at least for the young, the hardest part of it, what help to seek, and where and how to seek it, are no unimportant questions and in a practical treatise well deserve a few words.

Religion.—Far above all other assistance must, of course, be placed the influence of religion—not the superstition of which the bitter poet speaks:

> "Humana . . . cum vita jaceret
> In terris oppressa gravi sub religione,"

but that whose chiefest beatitude is promised to the "pure in heart."

Of the direct personal influence of religion upon the individual in this respect, it is not my purpose to speak here—the very nature of that influence is, in these days, the ground of too much and too fervid controversy. It is not, however, without interest to observe the different way in which the two great western divisions of the Christian Church treat the subject of continence.

Among *modern* Protestants, I cannot help feeling that there is, both in the spoken and written teaching of their authorized ministers, a certain timorousness in dealing with the matter, which, however natural, almost gives the idea of a lack of sympathy with the arduous nature of the effort requisite to obey the commands, that so urgently demand perfect purity from the consistent Christian.

It is much the same among the fathers of our Church. In those writings which are, from their antiquity, the wide assent they have commanded, the character and station of their authors, or from other causes, usually regarded as of *authority* among us, there is often a deficiency in frank and kindly discussion of the subject.

It was far from my intention, when I commenced this work, to put myself forward as a religious adviser, but I so frequently receive painful letters from young men, seeking advice how to

perfect purity, for those who would reap the blessings of continence.[1]

[1] "1. Of this commandment we can say but little. St. Francis de Sales says that chastity is sullied by the bare mention of it. Hence let each person, in his doubts on this subject, take advice from his confessor, and regulate his conduct according to the direction which he receives. I will only observe here in general that it is necessary to confess, not only all acts, but also improper touches, all unchaste looks, all obscene words, and whether they are spoken with complacency and danger of scandal to others. It is, moreover, necessary to confess all immodest thoughts. Some uninstructed persons imagine that they are bound only to confess impure actions; they must also confess all the bad thoughts to which they have consented. Human laws forbid only external acts, because men see only what is manifested externally; but God, who sees the heart, condemns every evil thought. 'Man sees those things that appear; but the Lord beholdeth the heart.' (1 Kings xvi. 7.) This holds for every species of bad thoughts to which the will consents. In a word, before God it is a sin to desire whatever is criminal in act.

"2. I have said *thoughts to which the will consents.* Hence, it is necessary to know how to determine when a bad thought is a mortal sin, when it is venial, and when it is not sinful at all. In every sin of thought there are three things; the suggestion, the delectation, and the consent. The *suggestion* is the first thought of doing an evil action which is presented to the mind. This is no sin; on the contrary, when the will rejects it, we merit a reward. 'As often,' says St. Antoine, 'as you resist, so often are you crowned.' Even the saints have been tormented by bad thoughts. To conquer a temptation against chastity, St. Benedict threw himself among thorns, St. Peter of Alcantara cast himself into a frozen pool Even St. Paul writes that he was tempted against purity. 'There was given me a sting of my flesh, an angel of Satan to buffet me.' (2 Cor. xii. 7.) He several times implored the Lord to deliver him from the temptation. 'For which thing thrice I besought the Lord that it might depart from me.' The Lord refused to free him from the temptation, but said to him, 'My grace is sufficient for thee.' And why did God refuse to remove the temptation? That, by resisting it, the saint might gain greater merit. 'For power is made perfect in infirmity.' . . . .

"3. After the suggestion comes the *delectation.* When a person is not careful to banish the temptation immediately, but stops to reason with it, the thought instantly begins to delight, and thus continues to gain the consent of the will. As long as the will withholds the consent, the sin is only venial, and not mortal. But, if the soul does not turn to God, and make an effort to resist the delectation, the consent will be easily obtained. 'Unless,' says St. Anselm, 'a person repel the declaration, it passes into consent, and kills the soul.' . . . .

"4. The soul loses the grace of God, and is condemned to hell, the instant a person consents to the desire of committing sin, or delights in thinking of

5

Training of the Will.—And now, leaving the religious aids to continence to those authorized to speak on the subject from that

the immodest action, as if he were then committing it. This is called *morose delectation*, which is different from the sin of desire. . . . . He who contracts the habit of consenting to bad thoughts, exposes himself to great danger of dying in sin—*first*, because it is very easy to commit sins of thought. In a quarter of an hour a person may entertain a thousand bad thoughts; and every thought to which he consents deserves a hell for itself.

"5. My brother, do not say, as many do, that the sins against chastity are light sins, and that God has compassion on such sins. What! Do you say that it is a light sin? But it is a mortal sin: even a sin of thought against chastity is a mortal sin, and is sufficient to send you to hell. 'No fornicator . . . hath inheritance in the kingdom of Jesus Christ and of God.' (Eph. v. 5.) Is it a light sin? Even the pagans held impurity to be the worst of vices, on account of the bad effects which it produces. Seneca says: 'Impurity is the foremost of the world's wickedness; and Cicero writes; 'There is no more heinous pest than the indulgence of uncleanness.'—St. Isadore has written; 'Whatsoever sin you name, you shall find nothing equal to this crime.'

"12. For those who are unable to abstain from impurity, or who are in great danger of falling into it, God has, as St. Paul says, instituted matrimony as a remedy. 'But if they do not contain themselves, let them marry; for it is better to marry than to be burnt.' (1 Cor. vii. 9.) *But*, some may say, *father, marriage is a great burden*. Who denies it? But have you heard the words of the apostle? It is better to marry, and to bear this great burden, than to burn forever in hell. But do not imagine that, for those who are unwilling or unable to marry, there is no other means but marriage by which they may preserve chastity. By the grace of God, and by recommending themselves to Him, they can conquer all the temptations of hell. What are the remedies? Behold them.

"13. The first remedy is to humble ourselves constantly before God. The Lord chastises the pride of some by permitting them to fall into a sin against chastity. It is necessary, then, to be humble, and to distrust altogether our own strength. David confessed that he had fallen into sin in consequence of not having been humble, and of having, perhaps, trusted too much to himself. 'Before I was humbled I offended.' (Ps. cxviii. 67.) We must, then, be always afraid of ourselves, and must trust in God that he will preserve us from sin.

"14. The second remedy is instantly to have recourse to God for help, without stopping to reason with the temptation. When an impure image is presented to the mind, we must immediately endeavor to turn our thoughts to God or to something which is indifferent. . . . .

"15. The third remedy is to frequent the sacraments of penance and eucharist. It is very useful to disclose unchaste temptations to your confessor. St. Philip Neri says that a *temptation disclosed is half conquered*. And should

point of view, let us consider whether there is not much practical
counsel to be given to the boy or young man who, having been

a person have the misfortune to fall into a sin against purity, let him go to
confession immediately. By ordering him, whenever he fell into sin to confess it immediately, St. Philip Neri freed a young man from this sin. The
holy communion has great efficacy in giving strength to conquer temptations
against chastity. The Most Holy Sacrament is called ' wine springing forth
virgins.' (Zach. ix. 17.) The wine is converted into the blood of Jesus
Christ by the words of consecration. Earthly wine is injurious to chastity; but the celestial wine preserves it.

" 17. The fifth remedy, which is the most necessary for avoiding sins
against chastity, is to fly from dangerous occasions. Generally speaking, the
first of all the means of preserving yourself always chaste, is to avoid the
occasions of sin. The means are, to frequent the sacraments, to have recourse to God in temptation, to be devoted to the Blessed Virgin; but the
first of all is to avoid the occasion of sin. ' And your strength,' says Isaias,
' shall be as the ashes of tow . . . . and there shall be none to quench
it.' (Isa. i. 31.) Our strength is like the strength of tow thrown into the
fire—it is instantly burned and consumed. Would it not be a miracle if tow
cast into the fire did not burn? It would also be a miracle if we exposed
ourselves to the occasion and did not fall. According to St. Bernadine, of
Sienna, it is a greater miracle not to fall in the occasion of sin, than to raise
a dead man to life. ' It is a greater miracle not to fall when one is in the
occasion of sin, than to resuscitate the dead.' St. Philip Neri used to say in
the warfare of the flesh, cowards—that is, they who fly from occasions—are
always victorious. You say: *I hope that God will assist me.* But God says:
' He that loveth danger shall perish in it.' (Eccl. iii. 27.) God does not
assist those who, without necessity expose themselves voluntarily to the
occasion of sin. It is necessary to know that he who puts himself in the
proximate occasion of sin is in the state of sin, though he should have no
intention of committing the principal sin to which he exposes himself. . . .

" 22. But let us return to the necessity of avoiding the occasions of sin. It
is necessary also to abstain from looking at immodest pictures. St. Charles
Borromeo forbids all fathers of families to keep such pictures in their houses.
It is necessary also to abstain from reading bad books, and not only from
those that are positively obscene, but also from those that treat of profane
love, such as certain poems, *Ariosto*, *Pastor Fido*, and all such works. O fathers!
be careful not to allow your children to read romances. These sometimes do
more harm than even obscene books; they infuse into young persons certain
malignant affections which destroy devotion, and afterwards impel them to
give themselves up to sin. ' Vain reading,' says St. Bonaventure, ' begets
vain thoughts, and extinguishes devotion.' Make your children read spiritual
books, ecclesiastical histories, and the lives of the saints. And here I repeat:
do not allow your daughters to be taught letters by a man, though he be a
St. Paul, or a St. Francis of Assisium. The saints are in heaven."—" Instruc-

made aware (as I have suggested he should be) of the ruinous effects of early impurity—is desirous of living a life of continence.

His object is—our object for him ought to be—to preserve a pure and healthy mind in a pure and healthy body. Judiciously directed training and exercise of *both* towards this definite object would, I am sure, in most cases, reduce the difficulty of living a chaste life to the minimum, and, indeed, render the conflict rather a proud and thankful sense of self-command than an arduous struggle.

The first requisite is, that power of the mind over outer circumstances which we call "a strong will." Without this resolute grasp of the intellect and moral nature, to direct, control, and thoroughly master all the animal instincts, a man's life is but an aimless, rudderless drifting, at the mercy of every gust of passion or breeze of inclination towards tolerably certain shipwreck.

It is a solemn truth that the sovereignty of the will, or, in other words the command of the man over himself and his outward circumstances, is a matter of *habit*. Every victory strengthens the victor. With one, long years of courageous self-rule have made it apparently impossible for him ever to yield. The whole force of his character, braced and multiplied by the exercise of a lifetime, drives him with unwavering energy along his chosen course of purity. The very word we have used—continence—admirably expresses the firm and watchful hold with which his trained and disciplined will grasps and guides all the circumstances and influences of his life.

Contrast with this man the feeble-willed; for him the first

tions on the Commandments and Sacraments," translated from the Italian of Saint Alphonsus M. Liguori, Bishop of Agatha, by a Catholic Clergyman, pp. 154–173.

Divest this advice from the peculiar coloring derived from the Church of the writer, and, for the priestly confessor, substitute reverently the ear of our loving Father who is in heaven, and of him who took our human nature upon Him in its completeness, that we might have no doubt as to His capability of sympathizing with us in all our troubles and infirmities—Protestanize its phraseology in short—and it would be difficult to find any more worthy of adoption.—W. A.

little concession, the first lost battle between the will and a temp-tation, is but the commencement of a long series of failures. Every succeeding conflict is harder because the last has been lost. Every defeat lessens the last trembling remnants of self-reliance. And at last, with the bitterest pain of all—self-con-tempt—gnawing at his heart, with no strength to say "I will not"—under the tyrannous dominion of foul passions, which all the good that is left in him abhors, the man slinks and stumbles towards his grave.

But, more than this, the steady discipline of the will has a direct physical effect on the body. The young man who can command even his thoughts, will have an *easier* task in keeping himself continent than he who cannot. He who, when physical temptations assail him, can determinedly apply his mind to other subjects, and employ the whole force of his will in turning away, as it were, from the danger, has a power over the body itself which will make his victory tenfold easier than his who, unable to check bodily excitement, though determined not to yield, must endure in the conflict great sexual misery.

Dr. Carter, in his "Treatise on Hysteria," makes some striking remarks on the effect of continual direction of the mind in pro-ducing emotional congestion of organs, which illustrate this view of the subject. He says (p. 13): "The glands liable to emo-tional congestion are those which, by forming their products in larger quantity, subserve to the gratification of the excited feel-ing. Thus, blood is directed to the mammæ by the maternal emotions, to the testes by the sexual, and to the salivary glands by the influence of appetizing odours; while in either case the sudden demand may produce an exsanguine condition of other organs, and may check some function which was being actively performed, as, for instance, the digestive."

He also relates a very remarkable example of the intensity of the emotional influence. "A lady, who was watching her little child at play, saw a heavy window-sash fall upon its hand, cut-ting off three of the fingers; and she was so much overcome by fright and distress as to be unable to render it any assistance. A surgeon was speedily obtained, who, having dressed the wounds,

sexual desire, I sallied out to take my exercise. I was victorious always; and I never committed fornication; you see in what
robust health I am, it was exercise that alone saved me." I
may mention that this gentleman took a most excellent degree,
and has reached the highest point of his profession. Here then
is an instance of what energy of character, indomitable perseverance and good health will effect.

The advice given by Carpenter in the fifth edition of his work,
p. 779, is as follows:—" The author would say to those of his
younger readers who urge the wants of nature as an excuse for
the illicit gratification of the sexual passion, 'Try the effects of
close mental application to some of those ennobling pursuits to
which your profession introduces you, in combination with vigorous bodily exercise, before you assert that the appetite is unre-
strainable, and act upon that assertion.' Nothing tends so much
to increase the desire, as the continual direction of the mind
towards the objects of its gratification, especially under the
favoring influence of sedentary habits; whilst nothing so effectually represses it as the determinate exercise of the mental
faculties upon other subjects and the expenditure of nervous
energy in other channels."

With reference to the vital importance of a strong, well-trained
will, we may also quote the valuable testimony of Dr. Reid:—

" Let us, as psychological physicians, impress upon the minds
of those predisposed to attacks of mental aberration, and other
forms of nervous disease, the important truth that they have it
in their power to crush, by determined, persevering, and continuous acts of volition, the floating atoms, the minute embryos,
the early scintillations of insanity. Many of the diseases of the
mind, in their premonitory stage admit, under certain favorable
conditions, of an easy cure, if the mind has in early life been
accustomed to habits of self-control, and the patient is happily
gifted with strong *volitionary power*, and brings it to bear upon the
scarcely formed filaments of mental disease. We should have
fewer disorders of the mind if we could acquire more power of
volition, and endeavor by our energy to disperse the clouds
which occasionally arise within our own horizon—if we resolutely

tore the first threads of the net which gloom and ill-humor may
cast around us, and made an effort to drive away the melancholy
images of the imagination by incessant occupation."

It should not be forgotten that this training of the will is not
without its immediate and sensible rewards. Without it, or at
least without some measure of it, those faculties of the mind on
the regular exercise of which our success in any pursuit, and in
fact our general intellectual advancement depend, cannot be
rightly cultivated. How absolutely essential it is for the attainment of real happiness, which depends so largely upon self-ap-
probation, has been already noticed.

Exercise and Diet.—It is not, however, sufficient to train and
strengthen the mind and will; the *body* must be subjected to a
regular and determined discipline, before the proper command
can be obtained over its rebellious instincts. And this discipline,
when properly carried out, will not consist in any violation of
the natural rules of health, but in a strict conformity to the hygienic regulations which science has proved must be obeyed
before real health and vigor can be ensured.

For instance, religious and mental discipline may be vastly
assisted by partial or total abstinence from fermented drinks and
exciting animal food. Experience teaches us that by merely
judiciously stinting the food of man in quantity and quality,
while, at the same time, the brain is kept in exercise and the
body fatigued, the animal instincts may be well-nigh subjugated.
I cannot, therefore, but believe, that a well-directed combination
of spiritual, mental, and physical training would secure, as nearly
as man may hope for, a perfect result. I lay stress upon the
words "judiciously" and "well-directed," because it is necessary
I should guard myself against being supposed to counsel a rash
or unscientific self-treatment. Much of the danger which has
always attended attempts at ill-directed self-maceration,[1] by fast-

[1] I am inclined to believe that many of the penances which ascetics in
former times set themselves—such as starvation, scourging, and exposure—
were the most potent means then known of restraining the animal passions,
and teaching the sufferers from them to control their feelings ; with the same
object we may believe that many a hermit shut himself out of the world in
order to escape the effect of female society. In the present day I am ac-

ing and purgatives, undertaken sometimes with a view of correcting corpulency and sometimes for mortification's sake, by religious enthusiasts, will as surely wait upon unscientific training to
continence. During the initiatory period, at all events, some
medical superintendence is desirable to decide when the process
should be commenced and how it should be graduated, what
amount of pressure may be put upon each constitution, when to
increase and when to relax it, what should be the nature and
extent of exercise, and the quantity and quality of nutriment
required to keep the system in true form and balance.

I am convinced, all other considerations apart, that were there
one or two days weekly set aside by all of us for extreme moderation in diet, public health and morals would be much benefited.
The writer who would rationally consider and popularize such
discipline, would be entitled to our thanks as a public benefactor.
At present, all healthy persons in anything like easy circumstances, eat and drink too much. Our over-eating is often attended visibly by the pendulous abdomen and lethargic frame,
and less obviously by depreciated mental energy, and what I
may term an artificial desire and imaginary increase of sexual
power. The dining, drinking, and sexual indulgence which are
practised with unvarying regularity by too many of our middle
classes who take little or no exercise, are acting as surely, though
perhaps slowly, against the *mens sana in corpore sano* of the
generation, as the opposite system I recommend of bodily labor
and organized abstemiousness[1] would tend to its maintenance.
So we come after all to the good old adage on the way to live
well—" On a shilling a day, and earn it."

acquainted with individuals who in former times would have become such
misdirected enthusiasts;—for human nature is little changed, although the
fashion of self-chastisement has gone out. There are self-made martyrs in
this nineteenth century, as there were in the sixteenth.

[1] The influence of food in modifying the process of development is seen in
a very marked form in the hive-bee. The neuters which constitute the majority of every bee-community, are really females with the sexual organs undeveloped, the capacity for generation being restricted to the queen. If the
queen should be destroyed, or removed, the bees choose two or three among
the neuter eggs that have been deposited in their appropriate cells, and

Healthy and Intellectual Employment and Amusement.—The passive means of abstinence from exciting causes are not, however, the only ones that must be employed in order to maintain that condition of self-restraining health which we desire to see in young men ;—an active hygiene is most essential. Exercise, gymnastics, regular employment, and all agencies that direct the energies of the growing frame to its increase and consolidation, and away from the employment of the reproductive organs, should be regularly used. I am convinced that much of the incontinence of the present day could be avoided by finding amusement, instruction, as well as recreation, for the young men of large towns. Every association or institution which encourages young men to desire to live virtually to consort with one another on the principles of purity and self-denial seems to be worthy of all support and applause. Such bodies of young men are of the greatest use even to those who do not belong to them. They insensibly modify the tone of young men's society. They all help to render vice, at least open vice, unfashionable. This I believe to be one of the many good results arising from the praiseworthy efforts which have now for some years been made by the various Young Men's Christian Associations, to raise the tone of thought and feeling among the middle-class youth of England. Most perceptibly beneficial results, too, have been produced by the institution of reading-rooms, instruction classes, gymnasiums and places for healthy recreation, where young men may pass their leisure hours in a cheerful, agreeable way, and be not only to a great extent withdrawn from temptation, but directly brought under those influences which

change those cells (by breaking down others around them) into *royal* cells, differing considerably from the rest in form, and of much larger dimensions ; and the larvæ when they come forth are supplied with " royal jelly," a pungent, stimulating aliment of a very different nature from the " bee-bread " which is stored up for the nourishment of the neuters. After going through its transformation, the grub thus treated comes forth a perfect queen, differing from the " neuter " into which it would have otherwise changed not only in the development of the generative apparatus, but also in the form of the body, in the proportionate length of the wings, in the shape of the tongue, jaws, and stings ; in the absence of the hollow on the thighs, in which pollen is carried, and in the absence of the power of secreting wax.

above all others lessen the force of that temptation. Every measure that provides healthy and rational occupation for young people—such, for instance, as the government classes for improvement in art, and the throwing open the Kensington Museum for evening instruction—is a step in the right direction, and must tend to realize the one great object of improving the morals of the people.

Much has been written during the last few years on the national advantages of the Volunteer movement. Not the least, in my opinion, of these advantages is the direct influence it has had in promoting continence among our young men, not only by the excellent effect which drilling has had on their physique and health, but by the vigorous and interesting occupation it has afforded them for mind and body. It affords a notable instance of the effect which a well-directed movement, judiciously carried out, can have on the rising generation. Much of the dissipation and libertinage of our youth has depended upon their having had literally nothing to do when their day's work was over. A pursuit which draws a man away from low society, and encourages him to spend his leisure in healthy and ennobling recreations among his equals, is most profitable to himself and his country. If the Volunteer movement had done nothing more than this, the parents of England would have had ample cause for supporting it.[1] Seeing as much as I do of the private life of young men in England, I can safely say that a healthier tone has sprung up among them of late, dependent, I believe, in great measure, on the love for athletic sports. In the course of years, I trust, it

---

[1] The physical advantages of the Volunteer movement have, of course, struck others besides myself. In a leading article in the " Telegraph " for November, 1861, I read the following observations, which are evidently based on sound reason: "The physical advantages of the rifle-training are also great. A man of loose life or careless habits cannot become a good shot; dissipation over-night does not give either the cool brain or the steady hand absolutely required. In fact, the 'training' and 'keeping in good condition' required for success in our public matches are, though less harsh, as absolutely needful as those required from oarsmen in the Oxford or Cambridge crews. With such a new national game, loved by young Englishmen, we need not despair of keeping up fully to the old mark the physical and moral manliness of our race."

will be found to have exerted a most beneficial influence on the morals of the country.

I have now, I think, discussed the chief aids to continence. If honestly used, they will, in most cases, enable a young man to conquer in the noble endeavor to obtain and keep the mastery over his passions during the most trying periods of his life. Nevertheless, I should belie my experience as a medical man if I were to represent this struggle as an easy one. It needs the whole energy of any man to succeed completely. No legitimate inducement, therefore, to the effort should be withheld. The greatest of all such inducements undoubtedly is the hope of early marriage; and this I would urgently press on the young, that the continent man is generally the energetic man, and that to the energetic man his trial is likely to be but temporary. He may fairly look forward to the time when he may think of marriage as the happy end to very much of the temptation which now requires so much anxious watchfulness, and even painful effort to subdue.

In the previous editions of this book I treated only of the religious, educational, and hygienic plans for enabling a young man to continue or return to a continent mode of life which were most efficacious, leaving the medical treatment to a subsequent part of the book. Now, however, I propose before going further to show what surgical means there are of assisting the youth in his struggles against the temptations of the flesh.

Experience has taught me that the several remedies already considered, however beneficial in the slighter cases and in those where the sufferers have strong wills, are by themselves perfectly futile in a large proportion of the cases of young men who have little or no determination and perseverance. It is to this class of young men that the medical practitioner can render most important service, more especially when gymnastic remedies alone have been relied on and failed. The examination of a large number of youths teaches me that the sufferers through continence labor under a peculiar sensibility of the reproductive organs. No one who has not closely investigated this subject can have any idea of the morbid sensibility which we meet with, both externally and internally. If, therefore, we would assist the youth in maintaining continence, we must first of all palliate or remove this nervous hysterical-like sensibility which almost invariably attends such cases.

There are patients who can hardly allow the air to blow upon, or the clothes to touch their sexual organs. Such sensitive persons are afraid of using cold water, they dread the most cursory examination, and declare it would make them faint. The proposal to pass an instrument almost produces a state of catalepsy. In all these cases it is not pain, but the dread of being hurt, apparently, which produces the suffering. Once an examination is submitted to and the confidence of the patient gained, the cure progresses most rapidly. In many instances this morbid irritability is confined to the skin, others only complain when the urethra is touched, or when an instrument passes over some particular portion of the canal, yet a second introduction of the instrument produces no inconvenience. When a surgeon has to treat such nervous patients as these he will not be surprised that previous hygienic precautions or the inculcation of moral restraints have not succeeded in preventing emissions. As soon as these local remedies have dulled the morbid sensibility of the sexual organs, the greatest advantage is at once derived from the moral and hygienic remedies.

In commencing the treatment of such cases the surgeon must evince some firmness of purpose or the patient will not submit. The medical man in his first essays must be satisfied with moderate progress. In a day or two the patient will often ask him to proceed faster than he is disposed to do, so satisfied is the sufferer of the benefit derived from the remedy. This simple local treatment will often suffice to cure the patient, but in more serious cases it may be necessary to employ instruments and use injections. These, however, will be more particularly alluded to in the chapter on spermatorrhœa, to which I must refer my readers.

I have mentioned in the chapter on Marriage that its consideration as the legitimate hope of the young man who desires to remain continent suggests several questions, on each of which there is some difference of opinion, and neither of which should be omitted from consideration here. I refer to *celibacy, early marriages* and *early engagements.*

When a young man is instructed for the first time (say, by a kind and judicious father), as to the nature of the new sexual sensations he feels within him, and is at once affectionately warned against dangers of which he has hardly suspected the existence hitherto, and urged to adopt the rational means for escaping or overcoming them, his first thoughts may naturally be—"Is it really good for me to spend many years of my life without indulging these instincts, which are, after all, according to nature? I have heard of the evils of celibacy, and yet I am urged practically to adopt it."

Before long, again, other and more difficult questions will arise. A pure and innocent affection awakes within him all that is best and noblest, and in the new delights he exults in having discovered a way of reconciling duty and inclination. He feels, and rightly, that the loyal and, so to speak, sanctified passion he rejoices in, is infinitely better than any illicit indulgences would be; and is, indeed, a preservation from them, more powerful than he had any idea of. May he not joyfully unite himself to the object of his choice, even in his early youth? May he not, at least, betroth himself to her, even though he must wait many years for marriage to crown his hopes?

On each of these questions I would say a few words before leaving this branch of the subject.

CHAPT. II.—CELIBACY.

The term "celibacy" is generally used to mean continence enforced on one who is of a fit age to marry. Continence in mere boys and very young men is not what we are now speaking of. Of course every rational person must be an advocate for celibacy, or rather, the strictest continence, in the very young, and will admit that the youth should not only physically abstain, but so exercise his will as not to allow his thoughts to dwell on sensual matters, if he is desirous of excelling in his intellectual studies.

I believe I have already mentioned the fact that in children strong sexual desires are often accompanied by and produce a dull intellect. In the adult it is often found that the inordinate exercise of the sexual organs frequently annihilates the intellectual faculties. It is an undoubted fact that we meet with a large proportion of unmarried men among the intellectual, and some of the ablest works have been written by bachelors. Newton and Pitt were single, Kant disliked women. "They do best," says Bacon, "who, if they cannot but admit love, yet make it keep quarter, and sever it wholly from the serious affairs and actions of life; for if it check once with business, it troubleth men's fortunes and maketh men that they can no ways be true to their own ends."

It was doubtless from such considerations as these that our ancestors ordained that fellows at the universities should remain single. Similar reasons probably had their influence in inducing the church of Rome to prescribe that their priests should take vows of celibacy.

Whether or not the Roman Catholic priest continues celibate does not much interest the English public; but whether fellows at the universities should be allowed to marry, has occupied a good deal of attention during the last few years.

A married resident at Cambridge, formerly a celibate fellow of a large college, has favored me with the following opinion on the subject:

"As regards the celibate life of college fellows, many most practical reasons exist in support of that rule. A brief statement must first be made concerning the object of college fellowships. Their object is not, as many imagine, to make a monastic society; still less to perpetuate an order of clergy who take a life-long vow of 'obedience, chastity, and poverty.' The main design of college fellowships is to assist young men who have talents but no money. In electing one of its members a fellow, the college has the aim in view of assisting a man of proved ability to fit himself without interruption for active service of

Church or State.   Just as a parent would make his son an allowance in order to help him in starting his chosen career, so does
the college give a fellowship, to make its best men independent,
while they are engaged in work or study leading to an honor-
able course of life, whatever that course may be.   And let it be
specially noted that only to men of limited means does the college give this advantage; no one can be elected a fellow if he
has already a *certain* income exceeding five hundred a year; no
one can continue a fellow if he afterwards become possessed of
such a *certain* income; in that case he vacates his fellowship *ipso
facto* without exception.   Again, by the general rule on the subject, no one can hold a fellowship for more than a limited number
of years—ten is about the average.   By the end of such a time
as that it is fairly assumed that a man will be ready to make his
own good way in the world, without requiring his college to help
him.   The fellowship was not given the man to make him ' idle
and affluent,' but simply in order to secure him the proper leisure
for 'working;' to save him the time he would otherwise spend in
earning his own bread.   As to 'affluence,' the average fellowship
never exceeds three hundred a 'year.   In days like these it is
but a bare provision, even for a man who has only himself to
keep.

   "The above statement will help to explain what practical reason the college has for strongly dissuading its fellows from marriage.   Would any parent advise his son otherwise?   If only
able to make him an allowance for some ten years, or a little
more, would not the parent warn his son on no account to marry
until he had secured his position?   Would not he urge him to
throw his energies, without distraction and without incumbrance,
into an earnest preparation for the actual work of life, and to
wait, at least, till he is turned of thirty before he thinks of in-
curring new responsibilities?   A young man with private prop-
erty can please himself in the matter of marrying early: but a
young man dependent on others, be those others his parents or
be they his college, is not free to please himself, but is bound in
moral duty to secure his own independence first before he thinks
of marriage.

"So far I have spoken of all fellows of colleges, whether they 'reside' or not; by 'residing' I mean 'living at the university.' Every fellow has the option of doing this if he pleases. Some of the liberal professions, e. g., divinity or physic, can be studied quite or nearly as well at the university as anywhere else; but, in point of fact, few fellows reside unless they have been appointed to hold collegiate office. And this brings us to another reason in favor of college celibacy. One of the objects of fellowships is this: to secure a class of superior men who will give their whole time and interest to the care of the college estates, to the management of the college itself, to the education of the under-graduates, and generally to the fulfilment of all academic duties. Of course a single man is able to do all this without interruption and with undivided energies; whereas a married fellow would be bound to bestow a part of his time on his family, would find his domestic interests often conflicting with his collegiate and aca-demical, would be unable to live within the college walls, which are quite unequal to such an accommodation; in fact, a married fellow would not be a person of the class which the founders of fellowships wished to keep established. That colleges would ever be managed without such a class of celibates is very doubtful indeed, and some of us would call it impossible.

"A third reason in favor of celibacy is that it somewhat in-creases the chance of fellowships falling vacant. Of course there are many fellows who marry within ten years of being elected; and if the celibate rule be maintained, fellowships then fall vacant with so much the greater frequency. This is the more desirable, because there are certain exceptional cases in which the fellow-ship can be retained beyond the limit of ten years. If a man be holding university office, or college office, or be in orders, he still retains his fellowhip although he has passed the limit. The reason is very simple; university office or college office, in point of money, is a mere pittance—no one could hold it without ad-ditional income; and the value of the man's college services is fairly considered a claim on his part to share, as before, in the college revenues, so long as he is actually serving: a non-resident has no such claim. As regards the profession of orders, it is so

6

cerned, that the old rule of celibacy has become a thing of the past, or at least it is so far tempered by modern changes and chances that no one now could esteem it 'a yoke too grievous to bear.' At Cambridge, no doubt, as elsewhere, 'persons intending to marry' must wait till time, position, and income all concur to endorse their intention. But looking on college office and college work as a profession, it cannot be denied that now it offers the same facilities for marriage as any other.

"Though I am one of the many who profit in some degree by these and the like alterations, I still retain my conviction that the old arrangement was best. Of this, at least, I am certain, that for college government a certain number of celibate fellows are indispensable. If all the college officers were married and living out of college, discipline among the undergraduates could not be at all maintained, and personal influence, close association, would all but cease to exist. Each college is at present a religious house, with the very highest standard of morality, and quite unrivalled facilities of education. And the real management of every college depends on the body of celibates who live within the walls and devote themselves to the work. Every change which, in any degree, diminishes the number of such collegiate authorities cannot but be more or less injurious to all our university system.

"I do not for a moment deny that celibate life involves a great self-sacrifice; but so does every human career which has high and noble aims. Surely the universities, like every other sphere in the country, will never fall short of men enough to fill up their posts of duty—posts which none but a celibate is really qualified to fill. There are always men in England (and an ample supply of such men) who have strength enough to forego the indulgence of physical and sentimental passion, when they know that by such self-denial only can their work be properly carried out. Nor do such men regard themselves, nor can we regard them as martyrs. College celibacy, at least, is anything but a martyrdom; to some well-balanced constitutions it is not a sacrifice at all, but purely a matter of preference. These are the men who persevere in retaining their fellowships twenty or thirty years,

instinct and passion within, but from the unworthy tone and example of friends and society without. I have come at length to believe that the drawbacks of collegiate celibacy are very much overstated. Indeed I venture to go further, and to say that at the universities themselves, these drawbacks, if they exist at all, exist in no perceptible degree.

" This is partly due to the fact that the life of a college fellow is intensely active and laborious. The real work of academic life *begins* only when the fellowship has been won. It would be difficult to find anywhere a body of men more constantly employed than the academic fellows, more versatile, more inquiring, more practical and energetic. For is there any class in England who receive so insignificant a payment for constant and serious exertion, Their healthful and regular employment which is scarcely ever sedentary, confers, however, its own reward; they have no time for self-indulgence, except in one good item, the practice of hospitality. It 'is a positive fact of any fellow at Cambridge that he is generally to be found in one or other of three distinct positions, either working his brain or else working his muscles, or else as a host or guest at table; all his amusements and recreations are of a vigorous 'gregarious' kind. Every. one knows what a marked effect solitude stamps on any constitution ; solitude at Oxford or Cambridge is the rarest of all conditions.

"Another fact which makes it easy to combine morality and celibacy is that, at either university, the men who remain as celibates are men of exceptional power, with nerve enough to be continent, with knowledge enough of life to know the value of such a regimen. Men with stronger animal and weaker moral nature rarely remain in a sphere like this, for which they feel unfitted; they make their way elsewhere, and soon vacate their fellowships; the problem solves itself, and the college gains by the solution. Celibacy serves as a wholesome test ; it keeps for college service the best and the strongest mind, excludes from college service the weaker, more sensual creature.

" If this conception of university life should seem to be formed on too exalted a scale, let readers remember that, as I have stated, the conception no longer is carried out to its full original extent.

In former editions of this book I made the assertion that in the adult the intellectual qualities are usually in an inverse ratio to the sexual appetites.

It has been pointed out to me that there are so many exceptions to this rule, that I have thought it necessary to modify the language in which I have expressed my views. I maintain that debauchery weakens the intellect and debases the mental powers, and I reassert my opinions that if a man observe strict continence in thought as well as deed, and is gifted with ordinary intelligence, he is more likely to distinguish himself in liberal pursuits than one who lives incontinently, whether in the way of fornication or by committing marital excesses. The strictest continence, therefore, in the unmarried and very moderate sexual indulgence in the married state, best befits any one engaged in serious studies. In making this statement, however, I am bound to admit that in practice we meet with a large number of young men of more than average abilites but of a delicate constitution, who cannot remain continent without becoming subject to frequent nocturnal emissions. When this is the case, the sufferer may be intellectually in a worse plight than if he were married and so occasionally indulged in sexual intercourse. In these exceptional instances it is not true that celibacy is the state best adapted to intellectual excellence. Of this I have had satisfactory evidences. Numbers of men studying at the universities come to me complaining that, although living a continent life, they have become so troubled by emissions that they are unable to pursue for any length of time hard or continuous intellectual work: their memories fail them, and their health becomes impaired. Under appropriate treatment the constitution rallies, and the intellectual powers are restored. From these and other cases that come under the care of the medical practitioner, it appears that celibacy in the adult is not unattended with danger to exceptional temperaments. These dangers, however, it should never be forgotten very seldom attend perfect continence. It will be generally found that they are merely the penalty of past indulgences. Robust, energetic men, are seldom troubled in this way—at least without some fault of their own. In all such cases

This opinion has been entertained by many excellent men; but if we examine it from a medical point of view, it is very doubtful, to say no more, whether it is desirable for any youth, who has his way to make in the world, to attach himself to a girl early in life, however purely and faithfully. If an adult is in a position to marry, by all means let him do so. If his sexual desires are strong, the power of the will deficient, and if his intellectual faculties are not great, early marriage will keep him out of much mischief and temptation. All medical experience, however, proves that for any one, especially a young and susceptible man, to enter into a long engagement without any immediate hope of fulfilling it, is physically an almost unmitigated evil. It is bad for any one to be tormented with sexual ideas and ungratified desires year after year. The frequent correspondence and interviews cause a morbid dwelling upon thoughts which it would be well to banish altogether from the mind; and I have reason to know that this condition of almost constant excitement has often caused not only dangerously frequent and long-continued nocturnal emissions, but most painful affections of the testes. These results sometimes follow the progress of an ordinary two or three months' courtship to an alarming extent. The danger and distress may be much more serious when the marriage is postponed for years.

I am aware that to the more romantic of my readers these warnings may be very distasteful. Their idea of love is that it is a feeling too pure and spiritual to be defiled with any earthly alloy. I confess that I doubt whether any but the inexperienced really entertain this notion. During the first passionate delight of an attachment, no doubt, the lower and more mundane feelings are ignored. But they are present nevertheless; and according to my professional experience, are tolerably certain to be aroused in every case sooner or late. Of course, where the affection felt is true and loyal, they may be corrected and kept within the strictest bounds of the most respectful tenderness; to do this, however, in the case of a protracted engagement is a far harder task than the ardent and poetical lover allows himself at first to think.

The suffering caused by the repression of continually excited feelings that cannot be gratified, is often very great.

I am very far from wishing to degrade love to mean animal passion; on the contrary, it should be a true and deep union of the whole nature, every part taking in this, as in all other matters, its own place. To ignore the bodily and secular aspect of it, however, would be as false and unwise, though not so degrading, as to forget the mental and spiritual.

It is, indeed, more than false and unwise, it is dangerous. Experience too often proves that what has commenced as a pure and most refined attachment may end very differently, if not most carefully guided. And this guidance, as I have said, may involve much troublesome and almost dangerous distress.

Continence from *all* sexual excitement in thought and deed is my advice to *all* young men; and even the adult, who is not in a position to marry, had better divert his thoughts from sexual matters as much as possible. It is wiser for him to devote himself altogether to his profession, and not have to divide his attention between a *fiancée* and his success in life. When the latter is attained, it will be time to think of the former. He will then be in a better position to select his partner for life.

Socially speaking, too, these long or early engagements often turn out badly. Hope deferred not only makes the heart sick, but the temper sour. Differences that the closer bond of marriage would have healed at once, or never allowed to arise, become permanent sources of disagreement, and very often the parties have to regret a youth that has been rendered less useful and less happy by an engagement which has at last to be broken off, after much suffering, to the mutual relief of both.

George Herbert says, in his "Church Porch:"

> " Wholly abstain, or wed—thy bounteous Lord
> Allows the choice of paths—take no by-ways,
> But gladly welcome what he doth afford,
> Not grudging that thy lust hath bounds and stays;
> Continence has its charms—weigh both, and so
> If rottenness have more, let heaven go."

In the case of *young* men, however, the rules above laid down apply with nearly equal force to early marriages. Lycurgus forbade any man to marry under the age of thirty—a state of celibacy probably well adapted to the times. As to early marriages I can only say that marriage, even for a boy, is better than fornication. But the true remedy, it cannot be too often repeated, for sexual distress in youth is a training to continence, not indulgence, even lawful. Those are in error who think that early marriages are advisable on the theory that there is no alternative.

After a pretty wide experience I should lay it down as a rule that marriage for the very young is not only not in any sense necessary, but is an evil, both from a medical and a social point of view.

No medical man, I hold, should ever recommend the hardly worked metropolitan population to marry *early*. Marriage is not the panacea of all earthly woes, or the sole correction of all earthly vices. It often interferes with work and success in life, and its only result is, that the poor man (poor in a pecuniary point of view) never reaches the bodily health or social happiness he might otherwise have reasonably expected. Under the age of twenty-five, I have no scruple in enjoying perfect continence. The sighing lackadaisical boy should be bidden to work, righteously and purely, and win his wife before he can hope to taste any of the happiness or benefits of married life.

PART II.

DISORDERS IN YOUTH.

CHAPT. I.—INCONTINENCE.

IN the previous chapter I spoke of the advantages of continence in youth. My remarks would not be complete were I to omit to say a few words on the evils of incontinence. I feel this to be all the more needful, as I am well aware that young

The medical, or so-called scientific adviser, who should recommend the commencement of a habit so dangerous, incurs the gravest responsibility. It should be rather the medical man's object to impress upon his patient's inexperienced mind the simple truth, that instead of being a mere sexual indulgence, the consorting with prostitutes is one of the very worst sins, both in nature and result, which man can commit. His tone should rather be that adopted in the following extract from a celebrated article in the "Quarterly Review:"

"Our morality will be considered by the divines as strangely lax and inconsistent, and by men of the world, the ordinary thinker, and the mass who follow current ideas without thinking at all—as savage and absurd; nevertheless we conceive it to harmonize with the ethics of nature and the dictates of unsophisticated sense. We look upon fornication, then (by which we always mean promiscuous intercourse with women who prostitute themselves for pay), as the worst and lowest form of sexual irregularity, the most revolting to the unpolluted feelings, the most indicative of a *low* nature, the most degrading and sapping to the loftier life,—

'The sin, of all, most sure to blight—
The sin of all, that the soul's light
Is soonest lost, extinguish'd in.'

Sexual indulgence, however guilty in its circumstances, however tragic in its results, is, when accompanied by love, a sin *according to nature;* its peculiarity and heniousness consist in its divorcing from all feelings of love that which was meant by nature as the last and intensest expression of passionate love; in its putting asunder that which God has joined; in its reducing the deepest gratification of unreserved affection to a mere momentary and brutal indulgence; in its making that only one of our appetites which is redeemed from mere animality by the hallowing influence of the better and tenderer feelings with which nature has connected it, as animal as the rest. It is a voluntary exchange of the passionate love of a spiritual and intellectual being for the hunger and thirst of the beast. It is a profanation of that which the higher organization of man enables him to elevate and refine. It is the introduction of filth into the pure sanctuary of the affections. We have said that fornication reduces the most fervent expression of deep and devoted human love to a mere animal gratification. But it does more than this: it not only brings man down to a level with the brutes, but it has one feature which places him, far, far below them. Sexual connection with them is the simple indulgence of a natural desire mutually felt; in the case of human prostitution, it is in many, probably in most, instances a brutal desire on the one side only, and a reluctant and loathing submission, purchased by money, on the other. Among cattle the sexes meet by common instinct, and a common will; it is reserved for the human animal to treat the female as a mere victim to his lust."—"Quarterly Rev.," July, 1850.

sexual abstinence, and so check population, they (mankind) have been willing to submit to the smallest proportion of food and leisure which the human frame could for a season endure. The want of love is so miserable a state of constraint, and, moreover, so destructive to the health of body and mind, that people who have a choice in the matter will rather put up with any evils than endure it.

*　*　*　*　*　*

"It may be mentioned as curious, that a young man entering on puberty is to indulge the exercise of all his organs, all his feelings, except that of the most violent—namely, love."

Few will be surprised, after reading the above, to find that this writer[1] feels himself obliged, for consistency's sake, to admit that what he calls *unmarried intimacy* should be sanctioned, precautions being taken to prevent the females having children; and to propose that the frail sisterhood should be received into society, because both they and their paramours but follow Nature's laws, and indulge sexual desires which Nature has given them for their own gratification.

I mention these opinions here, not with the intention of refuting them, but as showing the consequences such an argument must lead to, if carried out. I leave it to the reader's imagination to depict the state of society which would ensue.

Fortunately, such sophistry as that I have quoted is rare among English authors of reputation or ability. Similar sentiments, nevertheless, no doubt often float vaguely in the minds of many, especially in early life. The answer to them is very clear in the case we are now considering, viz. that of boys who have only just reached the age of puberty. For them it is sufficient to state the simple physiological fact, that, merely considering a

[1] The anonymous author when he wrote this dangerous volume was a medical student. Let us hope that ere this he has seen reason to alter his views, although, I regret to say, the latest edition of the work still contains these untrue and unphysiological statements. I presume it is from such evidence as is gleamed from this writer that Professor Newman, an Emeritius Professor of University College, has in a recent pamphlet taken the medical profession to task for recommending fornication—a charge which I wish most energetically to repel.

power can be properly exerted for the continuance of the race; and all experience shows that by prematurely and unrestrainedly yielding to the sexual instincts, not merely the generative power is early exhausted, but the vital powers of the organism generally are reduced and permanently enfeebled, so that any latent predisposition to disease is extremely liable to manifest itself, or the bodily vigor, if for a time retained with little deterioration, early undergoes a marked diminution."

One argument in favor of incontinence deserves special notice, as it purports to be founded on physiology. I have been consulted by persons who feared, or professed to fear, that if the organs were not regularly exercised, they would become atrophied, or that in some way impotence might be the result of chastity. This is the assigned reason for committing fornication. There exists no *greater error* than this, or one more opposed to physiological truth. In the first place, I may state that I have, after many years' experience, never seen a single instance of atrophy of the generative organs from this cause. I have, it is true, met with the complaint—but in what class of case does it occur? It arises in all instances from the exactly opposite cause—abuse: the organs become worn out, and hence arises atrophy. Physiologically considered, it is not a fact that the power of secreting semen is annihilated in well-formed adults leading a healthy life and yet remaining continent. The function goes on in the organ always, from puberty to old age. Semen is secreted sometimes slowly, sometimes quickly, and very frequently under the influence of the will. We shall presently see that when the seminal vessels are full, emission at night is not unfrequent. This natural relief will suffice to show that the testes are fully equal to their work when called upon. No continent man need be deterred by this apocryphal fear of atrophy of the testes from living a chaste life. It is a device of the unchaste—a lame excuse for their own incontinence, unfounded on any physiological law. The testes will take care that their action is not interfered with.

That continence is not followed by impotence is shown most forcibly in animals. Mr. Varnell, late a professor at the Veteri-

7

and exaggerations, until amidst the mass of error it is difficult for novices to detect the grain of truth which always lurks in popular belief.

When a youth has arrived at adolescence, I think he may, even by his parents or tutor, be fairly put into further possession of the information of what the sex-passion is—what the evils of its unchecked indulgence are—and what are the proper means to keep it within bounds.

CHAPT. II.—MASTURBATION IN THE YOUTH AND ADULT.

It will be convenient to discuss in this place the whole subject of masturbation in the youth and the adult, although it may be objected that it is not, strictly speaking, a *disorder* of the reproductive functions. It must be admitted that it is not a disease, although its effects are worse than those of most diseases. It is rather an habitual incontinence eminently productive of disease. However as the period of puberty is the time above all others when this scourge seizes its victims, it is as well to take this opportunity of considering it.

I purpose, also, as far as possible, to exhaust the subject here, so as to avoid any repetition of it under the head of " Disorders in Adults."

I have already, at page 24, in treating of the habit, as it is likely to affect children before the age of puberty, defined what it is ; and have included it in the definition of incontinence (page 52). I now proceed to point out what the results of masturbation are, when the vicious habit is practised after the age at which semen begins to be secreted.

It is often difficult to obtain much certain information on the subject during the early practice of the vice. Its unfortunate victims, so long as they can practice it with impunity, or are ignorant of its consequences, can hardly be induced to make the confession. A few authors who could avoid the task, have ventured even to speculate on the frequency of a vice at once so wide-spread and so deplorable.

"Soon taking courage, I learned that dangerous substitute which deceives nature, and saves young people of such a disposition as mine, from many disorders, at the expense of their health, of their strength, and sometimes of their life. This vice, which shame and timidity find so convenient, has, in addition, a strong attraction for lively imaginations. They have at their disposal so to speak, the whole female sex, and employ for their pleasure the beauty which tempts them, without the necessity of any avowal."—Edition Charpentier, p. 146.

If, to any reader, this description should seem too attractive to have been fitly inserted here, the next extract contains the antidote. None, I think, are likely to be fascinated by the Frenchman's vivid description of the *pleasures*, when he reads the equally vivid description of the *immediate* penalty of the abominable practice. No English youth with his eyes open would, I hope, willingly for any temporary gratification reduce himself to such a state of ill health as the French philosopher acknowledges he was suffering from.

The ultimate results, however, are the most terrible warning. With an astonishing mixture of blindness and sharp-sightedness, the misanthropic *philosophe* pries into his mental and moral character with a despicably morbid minuteness, apparently utterly unconscious that he has furnished a sufficient cause for the very tendency he thereby displays, as well as for the weaknesses and follies he laments over, and for the unmanliness, the pettish feminine temper and conceit, which would make a hearty English lad shudder with disgust, and which are only indications, after all, of lower and lower depths of mental and moral debasement.

He proceeds thus to describe himself, and presents us with what may be taken, after due allowance for self-deception and falsehood, for a tolerably accurate portrait of a masturbator half-way on the road to his ruin. The description is one of the most valuable and accurate I have ever read.

"One might say that my heart and my mind do not belong to the same person. . My feelings, quicker than lightning, fill my soul ; but instead of illuminating, they burn and dazzle me. I feel everything. I see nothing. I am excited, but stupid; I can-

all his life been able to learn six lines by heart. There are some of my sentences that I have turned and re-turned during five or six nights in my bed before they were in a state to be put on paper. Hence I succeed better in works that require labor, than in those which must be written with a certain degree of readiness, like letters—a kind of composition of which I have never been able to catch the proper tone, and the effort at which is misery to me. I never write a letter on the smallest subject which does not cost me hours of fatigue, or if I want to write at once what occurs to me, I can neither begin nor end; my letter is a long and confused veribage, hardly to be understood when read.

"But not only is it a labor to me to express, but also to receive ideas. I have studied men, and I think I am a tolerably good observer; yet I can see nothing of what I do see. I can hardly say that I see anything except what I recall; I have no power of mind but in my recollection. Of all that is said, of all that is done, of all that passes in my presence, I feel nothing, I appreciate nothing. The external sign is all that strikes me. But after awhile it all comes back to me. I remember the place, the time, the tone, the look, the gesture, the circumstance—nothing escapes me. Then, from what has been done or said, I discover what was thought, and I am rarely deceived.

"If I am so little master of my mind while alone, it may be conceived what I must be in conversation, where to speak, *à propos*, one must think at the same time and at a moment's notice of a thousand things. The mere idea of so many proprieties, of which I am sure to forget at least one, is enough to intimidate me. I do not even understand how a person can dare to speak in company—for at each word one ought to pass in review every one that is present; to be acquainted with all their characters and know their histories, in order to be sure to say nothing that can offend any. Certainly those who live in the world have a great advantage here; knowing better what *not* to say, they are surer of what they do say; yet even from them slips many an unfortunate speech. Imagine the condition of a man who falls into it all from the clouds; he can hardly talk

It would be well for humanity if masturbation did no more than produce even such humiliating mental effects as these. Daily experience teaches us that the evil habit is attended with the worst physical consequences also. These may as well be disposed of before we come to the last, worst, and most constant result, when the practice has become a confirmed habit.

At first we remark but little local irritation of the canal of the urethra. Pain may occur in making water, as well as a frequent desire to employ the bladder; the orifice of the meatus is frequently found red, and ejaculation, which before could only be excited by much friction, now takes place immediately; the secretion is watery, and even slightly sanguinolent, and emission is attended with spasm. A sense of weight is felt in the prostate, perinæum, or rectum, and anomalous pains are often complained of in the testes. Nocturnal emissions become very frequent, and are easily excited by slight erotic dreams. These at first are attended with pleasurable sensations, but later the patient is only aware of ejaculation from having his attention the next morning attracted to it by the condition of his linen. In other instances the semen does not pass away in jets, but flows away imperceptibly. In some cases it makes its way back into the bladder, to pass out with the urine. Other patients will tell you that emissions have ceased to occur, but on going to stool, or on the last drops of urine passing from the bladder, a quantity of viscous fluid, varying from a drop to a teaspoonful, dribbles from the end of the penis, which, if collected or allowed to fall on a piece of glass, and exposed to the microscope, may furnish spermatozoa in greater or less numbers.

The vicious habit having impaired the growth, health, and intellect of the patient, ceases often to be voluntarily indulged in, because pleasure is no longer derived from it. The drain on the system during defæcation or micturition, however, as I have stated above, continues, and what depended at first on an artificial excitement, is kept up by the irritation or inflammation of the urethra, vesiculæ seminales, and spermatic ducts. The too frequent irritation of the testes causes badly eliminated semen to be secreted, which is at once emitted. The mucous membrane is more sensitive than usual (see p. 77), acquires an irritability

tenance, the downcast expression, which seems to arise from the dread of looking a fellow-creature in the face, may be carried to the grave. Undoubtedly care and attention may do much in remedying the intellectual wreck which we notice in such youths.

It will be remembered that I am describing the results of only the worst and longest continued cases. The probability is that in many who read these pages and who have at some time or other practised this vice, but have early abandoned it, the symptoms will be of the slightest kind, and a speedy cure may be promised.

Quacks are eager, of course, to represent every case of the worst description; and I therefore wish clearly to guard myself against being supposed to mean that in my opinion all, or even most persons who have at any time fallen into this wretched habit are doomed to all the results above described. These results are, it is true, the end towards which sufferers are tending if they do not conquer the propensity, but if they do so before the last sad stage is reached, there is good hope for them yet. Nevertheless, the other extreme must be avoided, of thinking lightly of the habit, or denying that it is the cause of disease. A great change on the prognosis of these diseases has come over the profession in this respect of late, and many eminent surgeons now admit that various unrecognizable ailments are caused by these practices; and the "Lancet," in a series of remarkable leading articles, has recently (1870) suggested that all surgical authorities should discuss these ailments in the different manuals and dictionaries, instead of neglecting to treat of them as hitherto.

It is not very long ago that an able physiologist told me he believed that one half the boy population masturbated themselves more or less, and yet that the resultant consequences were very slight. He saw much of conscience-stricken young men who consulted him; but, in his opinion, they exaggerated their sufferings, and writers on the subject had magnified the ill-effects of self-abuse. This gentleman and those professional men who agree in this view have probably only met with slight cases, for there can be no doubt that there are others, whose wretched condition, mental and bodily, can hardly be exaggerated.

morbid feeling, it is the duty of the surgeon to assure his patient of sympathy and cordial help, and to do all in his power to remove these delusions.

Treatment.—In the earlier stages of this mental and bodily debility the services of the surgeon may be of great benefit. If a bougie be introduced into the urethra, and the treatment alluded to at p. 47 be employed, the patient will find it much easier to exercise self-control (which is what is wanted). If he will aid the surgical treatment, by taking gymnastic exercise and following the other rules laid down above, pp. 66, 74, a favorable result may be expected. It is in the earlier stages that relief should be sought, not when dementia has occurred, or when the brain has become disorganized. Those who treat mental diseases are not consulted sufficiently early to recommend this treatment; they see the effects when too often the mischief is irremediable; and it may be from the impression thus produced that sufficient weight has not been as yet given to surgical treatment in the incipient forms of insanity, brought on by this malady.

If, however, a patient will not attempt self-control, mental as well as physical, and if, instead of consulting a qualified medical man, hearing from him a statement of the consequences of the practice, strictly following out the treatment recommended, and giving up the vile habit, he should abandon himself to humiliation and despair, the downward course may be very rapid and fatal. When this frame of mind has completely got hold of a man, the step to insanity in its worst and most hopeless form is alarmingly short.

CHAP. III.—INSANITY ARISING FROM MASTURBATION.

That insanity is a consequence of this habit, is now beyond a doubt.[1] The subject has recently been thoroughly investigated

---

[1] The connection between insanity and extravagant sexual desire is alarmingly close, as appears from many modern investigations, especially with regard to the central portion of the cerebellum.

Deslandes has remarked that, "in proportion as the intellect becomes enfeebled the generative sensibility is augmented."

been going on; he has changed not only in manner but in appearance; he has become so peevish and irritable, so reserved in his conversation, so apathetic in manner, so slovenly in dress, so contradictory and so uncertain in his actions, so hesitating, first determining on one thing, and before he could execute that changing to some other course, and has shown such a want of self-reliance. That quite recently he has grown more and more apathetic, more slovenly in dress, paying less attention to cleanliness, and becoming slower in his actions; that he is now not only irritable in his temper, but is at times violent; that he does things by "fits and starts," is impulsive, deliberating long, and then suddenly hastens apparently to carry out his intention; and has become so stupid-looking and lost, and incapable of taking care either of himself or his business; and all this has occurred without any apparent cause, except it may be his 'studious habits.' At last he can be borne with no longer; he is unmanageable in a private house, and is obliged to be removed from his home.

GENERAL SYMPTOMS.—" On entering an asylum for the insane, especially if it be one receiving patients from the middle as well as from the lower class of society, there is one group of inmates which may arrest the attention of the visitor from the contrast presented to the excited persons around him, on the one hand, and to those who are convalescent on the other. Engaged in no social diversion, the patients of this group live alone in the midst of many. In their exercise they choose the quietest and most unfrequented parts of the airing grounds. They join in no social conversation, nor enter with others into any amusement. They walk alone, or they sit alone. If engaged in reading, they talk not to others of what they may have read; their desire apparently is, in the midst of numbers, to be in solitude. They seek no social joys, nor is the wish for fellowship evinced.

" The pale complexion, the emaciated form, the slouching gait, the clammy palm, the glassy or leaden eye, and the averted gaze, indicate the lunatic victim to this vice.

" Apathy, loss of memory, abeyance of concentrative power and manifestation of mind generally, combined with loss of self-

the inclination for repose more marked, and the sleep more natural and refreshing; the sensations of hunger and thirst are once more experienced; the secretions are more active; the cleanliness of habit is attended to; the dress is looked after; the obstinacy decreases, and gradually an inclination and the ability to converse, return, and at last, though slowly, the health of mind and body is restored. Such, in favorable cases, is the result, but it too often happens that convalescence is arrested, and that the condition of ordinary or chronic dementia becomes established, and with it the prospect of recovery diminishes."

RELAPSES.—"Remonstrate with these victims after they are received into an asylum, whilst reason is still not quite destroyed, and they will agree with your remarks. They will express their thankfulness that they have yet been spared some portions of reason; they will express their deep abhorrence of their conduct; they will shed the tears of apparent penitence; and yet the old habit will be relapsed into; and when they think that they are removed beyond control, will once again indulge in their self-destroying practice. The determination to conduct themselves in the pure course is wanting, and in this there is evidence of the pernicious energy-sapping cause.

"Few accidents are more capable of occasioning annoyance and disappointment to the physician, and none more calculated to excite his pity and regret, than to find the recovery he regarded as certain, marred and prevented, or delayed, by the preventible act of the patient himself. This cause of relapse is but little believed in, except by those who are intimately acquainted with the habits of the insane; but regarding it as possible, many an unexpected and unaccountable relapse can be readily explained. When any tendency to indulgence has been observed in the early stages of mania, the prognosis ought to be stated in well-weighed words. The fact of a patient, neither epileptic nor the subject of paralysis (although in young men the former is more probable), who when put to bed was progressing favorably, being in a lost or much confused state when he got up on the succeeding morning would be significant of some

8

thiness arise in such patients, and, under the impression that they have committed the unpardonable sin—have sinned against the Holy Ghost—and that a future world presents no hope of joy or happiness for them, as they are excluded from it by their past conduct, they frequently make attempts to terminate their own existence.   Such an act is occasionally incited by hallucination of the aural organ; but I have not found that suicide is so frequently to be traced to this, as in other cases of mental aberration depending on other causes."

SELF-MUTILATION.—"Another peculiarity of these cases is the tendency frequently exhibited to self-mutilation, and, as reports show, the attempts are not unfrequently successful.   Thus is indicated an unsound reasoning power, the visiting on the supposed offending organs the faults of the ill-regulated mind."[1]

As Dr. Ritchie states, the delusions in many instances assume a religious character, and hence it is that it is repeatedly found that the cause of the sufferer's condition is supposed to be religion.   The delusions of this class generally are of the melancholic character stated above: fears that eternal happiness is lost—that they have no hope beyond the grave—that they have committed an unpardonable sin—or that they are unworthy to live.

From the true cause of the mental condition of these cases

[1] I was recently called upon to sign a certificate, for a gentleman of high standing in his profession, who was himself willing to enter an asylum. His case was a very sad one, and exemplifies the ideas a patient, in this state, forms of his own ailments. His history, which, however, I gleaned from him with some difficulty, was as follows :—Early in life he contracted the habit of masturbation, nevertheless he married, and lived tolerably happily with his wife ; and his marital duties were performed, he assured me, in a satisfactory manner. He became, however, depressed, his conscience told him that he had done wrong in abusing himself early in life, and he determined as a punishment, that he would cut away the testes. This he effected,—the parts healed, and the patient entered an asylum, which he subsequently left. At the period I saw him, he was in what, I suppose, I may call a lucid interval. He still regretted most bitterly his early sins, and was satisfied that he had not been justified in mutilating himself. He was conscious that he was again losing his self-will, and felt that he ought to be watched, lest he should further injure himself (I was told he had attempted his life).—W. A.

not being understood, the meaning of these reproaches for past conduct cannot be comprehended; and it is easily explained why a young man of apparently blameless life making these self-accusations, is regarded by his friends as suffering from acute religious feelings, whereas remorse or fear has generally more to do with his condition than true religious impressions or conviction.

It is probable that many of those young men whose insanity has become developed through revival meetings, of which there have been several instances, would, on close inquiry, be found to be of the class now occupying our attention.

In some patients, rash and even criminal acts are the result of the idea that an atonement may thereby be made for the sin committed. The attempt to injure the genitals and similar extravagances often, I believe, arise from such insane fancy. While, on the other hand, extravagant masturbation, or the tendency to commit rapes or unnatural crimes, may be in some cases traced to the not less insane desire the sufferer feels to test, and prove to himself, or others, that he is not impotent.

TREATMENT.—The long extracts I have given from Dr. Ritchie's pamphlet may testify to the high value which I set on this acute observer's remarks on this disease; I differ from him, however, somewhat as to the prognosis and treatment, and am far more sanguine than he is of the success which may be anticipated from appropriate management.

Still, when deméntia has set in, I quite agree with Dr. Ritchie, that the case assumes a very serious form, and then it passes from the surgeon's care into the hands of those who attend to such cases. Kind care and domestic attentions are all that can be suggested to soothe the latter days of these victims of ignorance or vice.

In the last edition of this book diffidence on my part prevented my giving any positive opinion on this subject, and I preferred quoting the opinions of Dr. Ritchie, who had then recently published his pamphlet.

The experience I have gained during the last five years has induced me (while allowing the present chapter to remain) to give my personal opinion on this most important question, and I confidently assert that, at least in the earlier stages of dementia caused by self-abuse, the greatest service can be done to the patient. Even in the more confirmed cases of insanity arising from this cause, I should not be disposed to give up the hope of effecting a cure, instead of consigning them to confinement in a lunatic asylum, and I trust that my personal experience may induce those who specially devote their attention to mental diseases to give my plan of treatment, recommended at page 77, a fair trial. One thing I can confidently promise, that if my advice does not cure the confirmed case, it cannot do any harm. If it enable but one poor sufferer to be rescued from the madhouse, it deserves a trial, and I think my professional brethren will often find that it succeeds in what they have previously considered hopeless cases.

CHAPT. IV.—PHTHISIS ARISING FROM MASTURBATION.

The attention of physicians has been of late years directed to this subject. In the year 1862, Dr. Smith read a paper before the Med.-Chir. Society, entitled "A Statistical Inquiry into the prevalence of numerous conditions affecting the constitution in one thousand phthisical persons when in health." In this paper, he stated that 11.6 per cent. of the males had committed sexual excesses; 18.2 per cent. had been addicted to masturbation, and 22 per cent. had suffered from involuntary emissions. I can, from my own observations, fully corroborate his statements, though whether the phthisical cachexia is to be regarded as a cause or an effect of sexual excess I am not sure. Delicate constitutions, with a consumptive tendency, are often very susceptible of sexual excitement. They are consequently peculiarly liable to nocturnal emissions, and to the temptation to commit excesses. Coupled with this special tendency, there is often in such persons a high spirit, and a carelessness of consequences, which will not yield to any slight indisposition. It may, perhaps, often be, in such instances, as much the constitution which predisposes to excesses, as the sexual excesses which induce the delicacy of constitution. There can be, however, no doubt that these

tion.   In order to satisfy myself that these affections of the heart were not organic, I have met in consultation most of the ablest men in London, and we have come to the conclusion that these patients are suffering from functional diseases of the heart, and consequently the prognosis becomes much less serious, provided, as I stated in the preceding chapter, the patients will forego these excesses, and treatment is prescribed calculated to enable the patient to gain mastery of his will and to exert self-control. As soon as this power of exercising self-restraint is gained, the usual tonics, stimulants, and sedatives will exert the beneficial influence proper to them, though they may have been taken previously without any benefit.   It is in this that the advantages of the modern treatment for diseases of the heart consist, and the results achieved fully bear out my favorable prognosis of such cases.

THIRD PERIOD—ADULT AGE.

THE FUNCTIONS AND DISORDERS OF THE REPRO-
DUCTIVE ORGANS IN THE ADULT.

THE following pages will, for the purpose of greater clearness and conciseness, be divided into two parts. In the first I propose to enter on general considerations relating to the sexual condition of the adult, and in the second, to refer, with rather more minuteness, to the special constituent parts and necessary requisites of the sexual act, viz., *erection, ejaculation*, and *emitted semen.*

FIRST DIVISION.

GENERAL CONSIDERATIONS ON THE SEXUAL CONDITIONS OF THE ADULT.

THE commencement of *adult* life is a period in human existence less marked, perhaps, but not less real, and hardly less critical, than that of puberty. The general growth of the body is complete. The immature limbs of youth are hardened into the firm and elastic frame of the man. The mental powers should be at their highest. The will and judgment should command, and yet be enlivened by the remains of youthful energy and enthusiasm. And, which is more to our present purpose, the virile powers, whose existence commenced at puberty, now at last matured, should be fit and ready to be exercised in obedience to the Creator's command to "be fruitful and multiply."

At a period differing in every man's life—but occurring generally somewhere between twenty-five and thirty—he is conscious, if he have lived on the whole a chaste life, of a great change in those sexual tendencies of which he has been frequently conscious before. They are no longer the fitful fancies of a boy, but are capable, he feels, of ripening at once into the steady rational passion, or rather purpose, of the full-grown man. The natural longing is there still, but it is no longer towards mere sensual indulgence (it will be remembered that I am speaking of the *continent* man) but is deeply tinctured with the craving for wife—and home—and children.

Still, it is not to be denied, that however purified and fortified by these additional elements, the sex-passion in a healthy continent adult is very powerful; very different from the sickly cravings of the voluptuary, or the mad half-poetical desires of a boy, but requiring his utmost efforts to control, and his best wisdom to guide, when he is able at last lawfully to indulge it.

My object, at present, will be to discuss these sexual desires in the adult with a view to furnish, if I can, some hints and suggestions which may not be without their use, in enabling him to judge wisely, and decide rightly in some of the most important crises of his life.

PART I.

NORMAL FUNCTIONS.

First let us recall the real physical character of the sexual desires. "They are," says Carpenter, "in man, prompted by instinct, which he shares with the lower animals. This instinct, like the other propensities is excited by sensations, and these may either originate in the sexual organs themselves, or may be excited through the organs of special sense. Thus, in man it is most powerfully aroused by impressions conveyed through the sight or touch; but in many other animals, the auditory and olfactory organs communicate impressions which have an equal power; and it is not improbable that in certain *morbidly excited states of feeling*, the same may be the case in ourselves. Localized sensations have also a powerful effect in exciting sexual desires, as must have been within the experience of almost every one; the fact is most remarkable, however, in cases of satyriasis,

produce not only venereal erethism, but even the very act of ejaculation."

It is to be expected, that, at the time when the man is physically in the fittest state to procreate his species, nature should provide him with a natural and earnest desire, a stimulus, as it were to the commission of the act which he is now fully competent to perform, not only without injury, but often with positive advantage to himself. This physical condition is thus described in the 'Encyclopædia of Anatomy:'

" During the period of excitement, spermatozoa are becoming rapidly adult, the testicles and the ducts are full of semen, the individual is in the condition of a fish with a full milt, or a bird or stag with enlarged testes. He now instinctively seeks the society of women. Intercourse with females increases his excitement, and all is ready for the copulative act." (" *Encyclopædia of Anatomy,*" *Art.* "*Vesiculæ Seminales.*")

These, then, are the physiological conditions of the adult male. He feels that MANHOOD has been attained, he experiences all those mysterious sensations which make up what we call VIRILITY.

CHAPT. I.—VIRILITY.

Lallemand thus describes the normal condition of the healthy adult.—" Virility, derived from the Latin word, *vir,* a man, is the distinctive characteristic of the male; it is the condition upon which essentially depends the preservation of the species. Is this deep and moral sentiment the artificial result of education, of social *convenance,* of institutions, &c.? Certainly not! for it is identical in all men, among all people, it is even more energetic, or at least more potent among the least educated, and the least civilized. It depends then evidently on the instinct of propagation, the most powerful feeling of all, after that of self-preservation." (Vol. iii, p. 124.)

This feeling of *virility* is much more developed in man than is that of maternity in woman. Its existence, indeed, seems neces-

My advice to all young men above twenty-five, who are in good health, is, to marry as soon as their circumstances enable them to maintain a wife. Everything tends to prove that the moderate gratification of the sex-passion in married life is generally followed by the happiest consequences to the individual. And no wonder, for he is but carrying out the command of the Creator—"Be fruitful and multiply, and replenish the earth"—in the way appointed by the Almighty Himself.

HINDRANCES TO MARRIAGE, REAL AND IMAGINARY.—It is a great misfortune, and a cause of much evil, that in our present state of *civilization*, the means of maintaining a family are so difficult of attainment as, in the case of certain classes, very much to restrict the power of fulfilling the above command, or of enjoying the privileges attendant on obedience to it.

It would be well if competent medical men who are called upon to give their opinion on this question of marriage, were only met by the difficulties of narrow means or the fear of having a large family. Many men are sorely distressed by forebodings, which can only arise from an ignorance that to the general public may seem hardly credible. In many instances it is a previous bad life which is the real source of most of the timorous unwillingness to marry. Few persons, perhaps, come into contact with so many conscience-stricken young men as I do. A youth who has abused himself, as soon as he learns the consequences, becomes alarmed, and sets down all his subsequent ailments to the particular cause which is ever uppermost in his thoughts, and his principal cause of disquietude is that he is unfit for the married state.

Among the most frequent consequences of this hypochrondriacal feeling, is the suspicion that he may not be able to consummate marriage. As this is a very common fear, and as, moreover, the vaguest notions exist among young men about marital duties, perhaps I may state that, as a matter of fact, there are comparatively few adults who would be really unable to consummate maraiage. The symptoms indicating a condition of real impotence will be fully given in subsequent pages, and of course those who really suffer in this way could never be advised

serve as an indication of this primary requisite, or of its absence. The existence of insanity or consumption in her family to any serious extent, should warn him, for his own sake and the sake of the children he might have, not to run the really terrible danger of marrying a woman whose family labor under either of these serious affections.

No one, it may safely be said, who has been habitually ailing during her girlhood, will make a good wife. Nay, I would carry the rule farther, and warn my prudent readers that *pale* women with colourless faces and waxy skins, even if they are tolerably strong themselves, very seldom have healthy children. So important is it to select for a future partner for life, and mother of children, a woman of undoubted health, that I even go one step further, and urge the man who consults me on such a subject, if he were free to choose, to select a *country* wife, especially if he himself be necessarily a dweller in a large town. The children of parents who are both Londoners are especially difficult to rear, so much so indeed, that some lay it down as a rule that, after three generations, every family that has uninterruptedly been born, lived and died in town becomes entirely extinct.

If a man be himself fair, I should advise him not to choose as a wife a women with flaxen hair, let him rather select a brunette. We often notice that parents, both of whom have light colored hair, beget scrofulous children, particularly if there be, as is often the case, a latent hereditary predisposition on either side, although no actual disease may exist in either parent.

Closely connected with the question of health is that of *education* and past history. It is probably almost unnecessary to urge men to avoid, if possible, a vulgar or bad-tempered mother-in-law. But it should not be forgotten, in the natural desire to escape unpleasant relations, that a member of a large family will, *primâ facie*, make a healthier, and sweeter-tempered wife, than an only child. As to intellect, accomplishments, and fortune, men need little advice. Literary women are not likely to be much sought after for wives. And great accomplishments so seldom survive the first year of married life, that men of the world are too sensible to allow them to outweigh the sterling qualities of a pleasant manner, a sweet temper, and a cheerful disposition.

As to *fortune*, it is hardly my province as a medical man to advise on this subject. Still I would suggest that, if the previous course of life which I have pointed out as best, has been really followed; that is, if a young man has lived a thoroughly continent life, in body and mind, until he is in a position to maintain a wife, there seems little reason in choosing his partner, to give the question of fortune any great weight. Most women will spend the fortune they bring, and the propriety of the husband's supporting, rather than being supported by his wife, as tending to make the home happier, is obvious.

As to *rank and position* in society, it is of course desirable that the wife should be selected as nearly as possible from the same rank of society as her husband. But if there is to be a difference, the husband ought, I think, to select a wife from a class rather above him. Men can and often do rise from a humble origin to a social status far above that of their wives, however great the disparity was originally. But this is very seldom the case as regards women. They generally maintain to the end *socially* the same as they were born. Money and a husband's position may do much, but it can hardly raise a vulgar, low born, or originally immodest woman one step in the social scale, however great her husband's fortune and position may be, or however faultless her own married life. She may, perhaps, to a certain extent, hide the traces of her early training from *men*, but her own sex, whom she meets in the rank of her husband's society, will be sure to detect them at once.

I have been often asked, "Shall I (other things being equal) marry for beauty?" I answer, "Yes, if you can get your beauty to accept you." Let ugly people talk as they may about intellect and the evanescent charms of mere outward comeliness, still some degree of beauty is, if not the first, certainly the second requisite in most cases, to a happy married life.[1] A tolerably large

[1] "How exquisitely absurd, to tell girls that beauty is of no value, dress of no use! Beauty is of no value; her whole prospects and happiness in life may often depend upon a new gown or a becoming bonnet; and, if she has five grains of common sense, she will find this out. The great thing is to teach her the just value, and that there must be something better under the bonnet than a pretty face, for real happiness. But never sacrifice the truth." — *The Rev. Sidney Smith.*

acquaintance with the domestic histories of men, in all ranks of life, has shown me that next to a good disposition, nothing in a wife is so likely to ensure domestic happiness as good looks, especially if they are of a lasting kind, not mere bloom or prettiness. We all must acknowledge that good looks are among the best passports in the world. Even children, the most unprejudiced witnesses possible, frankly admit that they like so and so, because she or he has a nice face. It is unwise to undervalue, or pretend to undervalue, the women's advantages of comeliness of face and form. A woman with a good physique starts with advantages that other women cannot acquire. She is spared a thousand and one temptations—jealousy and other low feelings supposed to haunt occasionally the female breast—with which her less favored sisters have to contend. Physical attractions, again, help to tide over many of those little domestic differences which will occur in married life. Man's sexual sense will be aroused by beauty when all other influences have failed to move him. It would be a curious inquiry, perhaps worth pursuing, whether, even among the lower classes, a comely-looking woman was ever ill-used by her husband, except when he was drunk. In a state of nature we find that animals select the most perfect forms for their mates—thus instinctively providing for the perpetuation of as perfect a species as possible. It would be well in many respects if this example were more closely followed by human beings.

That I do not exaggerate the importance of bearing these and similar considerations in mind in choosing a wife is tolerably self-evident. I may, however, refer those who require an authority to the Republic and the New Atlantis, to show what minute care Plato and Bacon recommended, in their ideal commonwealths, in the selection of those who were to be mothers and nurses of the citizens.

I have submitted the above remarks to a clever unmarried woman, and she has favored me with several additional observations on the subject, of which I gladly avail myself.

Almost the first thing a girl is told in the nursery is that beauty soon fades, and that ugly girls are as much valued as handsome ones; but on their first step over the threshold into the world a woman soon discovers the fallacy of this early teaching; and I perfectly agree with Sydney Smith in his remarks upon personal beauty as affecting the destiny of women. Comeliness of form and beauty of feature ought not to be despised, as they are the gifts of God.

Milton represents Eve as the embodiment of female loveliness. Sarai, the wife of Abraham, was a fair woman to look upon; and Rachel, Jacob's best loved wife, "was beautiful and well favored."

It is, however, very difficult to define in what beauty consists. It is more a kind of pleasure conveyed to the mind of the beholder than any special personal attraction of form or figure. All nations and ages agree in worshipping beauty of some sort or other. We see it portrayed in pictures and statues; and one of the great reasons for supposing that it is considered desirable in the eyes of man is, that where it does *not* exist women frequently try to supply its place by artificial means. It is said that Madame de Stael would have given up all her fame and renown to have been as beautiful as her friend Madame de Rocca; and I doubt very much whether we should have felt the same degree of pity for Mary Queen of Scots had she been as ugly as her illustrious rival Elizabeth.

It is, however, rare to meet with *very* ugly women. A mere set of features, however beautiful in form, seldom please an educated man, unless they are lighted up by good sense and good temper. A man soon gets tired of the pretty child wife. After twenty-five the bloom of youth begins to fade, and yet what is called *beauty* often lasts for years; so that, in a general way, it is the mind and morals that in a great measure influence the appearance of women and heighten their attractions in the eyes of men; and however much they may deny it, or try to conceal it, yet I believe there is inherent in every woman's heart a wish to be pleasing and agreeable to the other sex; and as it is in a great measure the destiny of most women to be married, it seems incumbent upon parents to give girls that judicious training in early life which will fit them to be good wives and mothers; and there is, I believe, no greater happiness on earth than is to be found in the married state, where two persons of affectionate dispositions, and equals in birth and station, agree to pass the rest of their lives together, till, in fact, death, and not Lord Penzance, them do part. In the higher grades of life beauty is often a binding tie; in the lowest ranks of life I do not think men deem personal appearance of any consequence. Much of the happiness in wedded life depends mainly upon the *woman*. She should be the sharer of his joys and the comforter in his griefs. She was made for him, not he for her; and her privileges as his companion are great and many. Now what kind of woman, in a general way, is most capable of heightening his joys and lessening his sorrows?

Sir Lytton Bulwer has summed up what a man wants in a wife. He wants a *companion*. "He does not want a singing animal, nor a dancing animal, nor a drawing animal,— and yet these three last accomplishments have cost many women years of painful toil to acquire; and they often marry a man who cannot appreciate any one of them." After forty, few women can sing, and few care to dance. A great proficiency in these accomplishments often leads a woman into expensive and dangerous society, where her vanity is fed by excessive praise.

What a man looks for most in the chosen companion of his heart and home is that she should have, added to a pleasing exterior, a well cultivated mind. Let her have also the "mens sana in corpore sano," good health and good temper; for what we call *happiness* depends very much upon the temper, and state of the digestion,—much more so, I believe, than we are generally aware of. Avoid marrying, if possible, a woman of an *hysterical* temperament. A few tears may be very interesting during that treacle period called the honeymoon; but in after life there is no misery for a man greater than to be united to a woman of delicate fibre and weak digestion, who, upon all occasions and no occasion, throws herself into that incurable and misery-causing malady,—a fit of hysterics. In early life it may be cured, but if suffered to go on for any lengthened period, it causes the patient to be a curse instead of a blessing to all connected with her.

I perfectly agree with you in the opinion that literary ladies do not generally make good wives, although, of course, there are exceptions. Their time and thoughts are too much engrossed by studies needful for their profession, to allow them to devote their time and thoughts to the daily comfort and well-being of their husbands. What Mrs. Hemans calls the dinner-ordering cares of life, are often neglected by authoresses. I *totally differ* with you in your opinion, viz., that if there is to be a difference in rank *husband* ought to be the lower. A woman sinks to the level of the man she marries. *He* can raise her, but she never can, and never does, raise him. Her pliant nature and yielding disposition accommodate themselves to his status in life; but I think such marriages are productive of very little happiness.

It seems a hard and unchristian opinion that it is better not to marry the daughter of a divorced woman; but I believe that the sin of unfaithfulness is often inherited, as well as many other family diseases.

The poet Cowper says, "that it is a wholesome rigor in the main, that, by the loss of chastity, women lose their place in the social circle; though—

> "It seems hard for here and there a waif
> Desirous to return, but not received!"

The pretty horsebreaker may be a pleasant companion in Rotten Row; but I much fear that, as a wife, she may end in breaking her husband's heart.

The French say that an Englishwoman makes a better mother than she does a wife, and they have some reason for so saying; as we often see, after the first year of married life a woman becomes a slave to the nursery duties and neglects her husband and her personal appearance; and, in fact, sinking the duties of wife into those of the mother, and often regarding the husband as an incumbrance instead of treating him as the *chief*, the real, the only one requiring her care and love.

But, after all, men must remember that women have many sorrows and much suffering to contend with, peculiar to themselves. The small cares and domestic troubles of life fall largely upon them, and they require much love

with which even the wildest male will approach the tame female when in heat, it would seem that no pleasure is equal to this.[1] There is every reason to believe that it is the mere and single act of emission which gives the pleasurable sensations in animals which (like many birds) have no intromittent organ. This pleasurable sensation, however, is of momentary duration; like a battery, it exhausts itself in a shock. The nervous excitement is very intense while it lasts, and, were it less momentary than it is, more mischief would probably result from repeated acts than ordinarily happens.

Parise has remarked, perhaps with some exaggeration, that "if the pleasurable moments, as well as the torments, which attend

[1] I am speaking here, it will be observed, of the pleasure experienced by the male. In the females of many animals, and especially of those low down in the scale of existence, we can scarcely believe that any gratification at all attends the act.

In fishes copulation, properly speaking, does not take place. According to Mr. Walsh, a close observer who wrote an account in the "Field" newspaper for March 7th, 1863, the mode of impregnation is as follows:—"The female fish does not first deposit her spawn, and then leave it to be impregnated by the male; the male cares nothing for the spawn, except to eat it; his desire is for the female, for the possession of whom he will fight as long as he is able. The spawning process is carried on in this manner:—The female works away at the ridd, and after she has made a kind of trough she lies in it quite still; the male, who during, the time she is working, is carrying on a constant war—comes up, enters the trough, and lies side by side with the female; then they fall over on their sides, and with a tremulous motion the spawn and milt are exuded at the same instant. The male then drops astern. After a short time the female again throws herself on her side, and fans up the gravel, advancing the trough a little, and covering up the deposited spawn. The operation is repeated till both fish are exhausted. A great quantity of spawn is of course wasted, being eaten by trout and other fish, which are always waiting about for the purpose. The exhaustion of the males is greater than that of the females; they die in numbers; the females do not die. You may pick up a great many exhausted and dead males, but never a female.

In some animals the act must, we would think, be an unmitigated distress, and annoyance to the female. The female frog, for instance, is not only encumbered with an abdomen distended with ova, but is obliged to carry about her husband on her back as long as he may see fit, as he is provided by nature at this period with an enlarged thumb, which enables him to keep his hold, so that the female is unable to shake him off.

love lasted, there would be no human strength capable of supporting them, unless our actual condition were changed."

A kind of natural safeguard is provided against the nervous exhaustion consequent on the excitement of coitus, by the rapid diminution of the sensation during successive acts. Indeed, in persons who repeat coitus frequently during the same night, the pleasurable sensation will diminish so rapidly that the act at last will not be attended with any.

This pleasure, in fact, seems, in its own way to be subject to the same laws which apply to our other gratifications. As Carpenter says—" Feelings of pleasure or pain are connected with particular sensations which cannot (for the most part, at least) be explained upon any other principle than that of the necessary associations of those feelings by an original law of our nature with the sensations in question. As a general rule, it may be be stated that the *violent* excitement of *any* sensation is disagreeable, even when the same sensation in a moderate degree may be a source of extreme pleasure."

By this merciful provision nature herself dictates that excesses must not be committed. The frequent complaint heard from persons who have committed excesses, that they experience no more pleasure in the act, is the best evidence we can have that nature's laws have been infringed.

The physiological explanation of the pleasure attendant on the sexual act is, perhaps, as follows:—"Accumulation of blood," says Köebelt, " causes, whenever it occurs in the body, a gradual augmentation of sensibility ; but in this case the glans penis, in passing from a non-erect state to the condition of complete turgescence, becomes the seat of a completely new and *specific sensibility*, up to this moment dormant. All the attendant phenomena react on the nervous centres. From this it appears that, in addition to the nerves of general sensibility, which fulfil their functions in a state of repose and also during erection, although in a different manner, there must be in the glans penis, *special nerves of pleasure*, the particular action of which does not take place except under the indispensable condition of a state of orgasm of the glans. Moreever, the orgasm once over, the nerves return to their former state of inaction, and remain unaffected under all ulterior excitement.

"They are, then, in the same condition as the rest of the generative apparatus; their irritability ceases with the consummation of the act, and, together with this irritability, the venereal appetite ceases also to be repeated, and to bring about the same series of phenomena at each new excitation."—*Köbalt,* "*Die männlichen und weiblichen Wollust-Organe des Menschen und einiger Säugethiere,*" p. 35.

Many foreign writers maintain, what the above observations would seem to corroborate, viz., that the chief source of sexual pleasure resides in the glans penis. That it has a considerable share in the sensations experienced is very true, but from certain cases that have come under my notice, I cannot help thinking that it has less to do with them than is generally supposed. Some time ago I attended an officer on his return from India who had lost the whole of the glans penis. This patient completely recovered his health, the parts healed, and a considerable portion of the body of the penis was left. I found, to my surprise, that the sexual act was not only possible, but that the same amount of pleasure as formerly was still experienced. He assured me, indeed, that the sexual act differed in no respect (as far as he could detect) from what it had been before the mutilation.

Duration of the Act.—It is probably well, as has been noticed, that in the human being the act should last but a short time—some few minutes.

In animals the greatest differences in this particular take place.

Thus I read in the "Description of the Preparation of the College of Surgeons," that "the coitus in the kangaroo, and probably in other marsupials, is of long duration, and the scrotum during that act disappears, and seems to be partially inverted during the forcible retraction of the testes against the marsupial bones.—No. 2477, *Physiological Catalogue, by Owen.*

The act of copulation as I have observed it in the moth of the silk-worm is very prolonged. The male is the smaller and darker of the two, and as soon as he leaves the grub state he is ready for the act. He then vibrates his wings with a very sin-

This nervous orgasm is very powerfully exhibited in some animals. The buck rabbit, for instance, after each sexual act, falls on his side, the whites of his eyes turn up, and his hind legs are spasmodically agitated. The cause of this, and the corresponding phenomena in other animals, is the nervous shock which particularly affects the spinal cord.

The way in which this shock affects a healthy man is, generally, to make him languid and drowsy for a time.

This temporary depression has not escaped the observation of the ancients, who have remarked—

> " Læta venire Venus tristis abire solet ;"

and again—

> " Post coitum omne animal triste, nisi gallus qui cantat."

So serious, indeed, is the paroxysm of the nervous system produced by the sexual spasm, that its immediate effect is not always unattended with danger, and men with weak hearts have died in the act. Every now and then we learn that men are found dead on the night of their wedding, and it is not very uncommon to hear of inquests being held on men discovered in houses of ill-fame, without any marks of ill-usage or poison. The cause has been, doubtless, the sudden nervous shock overpowering a feeble or diseased frame.

However exceptional these cases are, they are warnings, and should serve to show that an act which *may* destroy the weak should not be tampered with even by the strong.

Lallemand well describes the test which every married man should apply in his own case :—" When connection is followed by a joyous feeling, a *bien être général*, as well as fresh vigor; when the head feels more free and easy, the body more elastic and lighter ; when a greater disposition to exercise or intellectual labor arises, and the genital organs evince an increase of vigor and activity, we may infer that an imperious want has been satisfied within the limits necessary for health. The happy influence which all the organs experience, is similar to that which follows the accomplishment of every function necessary to the economy."

How serious—how *vital* an act, so to speak, that of copulation is, appears from the marked changes which accompany its performance in some animals. It is a well accredited fact that in the rutting season buck venison is strong, lean, and ill-flavored. At this time, we are told, the flesh becomes soft and flabby, the hair looks "unkind;" and in birds, the feathers, after the season of breeding, are in a ruffled state, and droop. The horns of stags (see Chapt. III.—The Emitted Semen) fall off, and the blood is occupied in supplying the consequent demand for new osseous matter.

It is before the spawning season has passed that we prefer the herring, and it is only while it is filled with roe, that we care to eat the mackerel. A spent salmon is not fit food for man; and, at this period, as all fishermen are aware, the vivid colors of the trout disappear; and the fish retires exhausted and impoverished, until the vital forces are regained.

Repetition of the Act.—Whilst one individual will suffer for days after a single attempt, or even from an involuntary emission, another will not evince the least sign of depression, although the act is repeated several times in succession or on several consecutive nights. Still, as a general rule, the act is and ought to be repeated but rarely. In newly married people, of course, sexual intercourse takes place more frequently, and hence it happens that conception often fails during the first few months of wedlock, depending probably upon the fact that the semen of the male contains but few perfect spermatozoa: in such cases it is only when the ardor of first love has abated, and the spermatozoa have been allowed the time requisite for their full development, that the female becomes impregnated.

This part of my subject will, however, occupy further attention when I come to speak (page 148) of marital excesses. I may, however, here state that the monthly periods, of course, put a stop to the act, while nature provides a kind of check upon its too frequent repetition, in the effect which pregnancy produces on the female, and through her upon the male.

If the married female conceives every second year, we usually notice that during the nine months following conception she experiences no great sexual excitement. The consequence is that sexual desire in the male is somewhat diminished, and the act of coition takes place but rarely. Again, while women are suckling there is usually such a call on the vital force made by the organs secreting milk that sexual desire is almost annihilated.[1] Now, as experience teaches us that a reciprocity of desire is, to a great extent, necessary to excite the male, we must not be surprised if we learn that excesses in fertile married life are comparatively rare, and that sensual feelings in the man become gradually sobered down.

It is a curious fact that man and a few domesticated animals are alone liable to suffer from the effects of sexual excesses. In a state of nature wild female animals will not allow the approach of the male except when in a state of rut, and this occurs at long intervals and only at certain seasons of the year. The human female probably would not differ much in this respect from the wild animal, had she not been civilized, for as I shall have occasion again and again to remark, she would not for her own gratification allow sexual congress except at certain periods. The courtezan who makes a livlihood by her person may be *toujours pres*, but not so the pregnant wife or nursing mother. Love for her husband and a wish to gratify his passion, and in some women the knowledge that they would be deserted for courtezans if they did not waive their own inclinations may induce the indifferent,

---

[1] We are apt to believe that in the human female it is almost impossible for gestation and lactation to go on simultaneously. In the mare, however, this occurs. In large breeding establishments the mare is usually put to the stallion, and will "show to the horse" nine days after a foal is dropped. The object of this of course is that in eleven months she shall again give birth to another foal. This is the surest way to obtain foals, although the produce of a mare after being a year barren is generally stronger and presumably better than on her becoming with foal while suckling. In fact, if left a twelvemonth barren, mares, I am informed by competent men, are stinted with great difficulty.

Mr. Blenkiron, the well-known breeder of race horses at Middle Park, has kindly looked over this note, and he tells me that, although this happens, mares often require some little management " to show to a horse, although in season," and it is necessary to put the twich on the nose to distract their attention, otherwise their affection for the foal induces them " not to show to the horse, although in season."

ought to be, always limited to a certain number of mares, but as he takes his mounts during a limited time (two or three months), the act is necessarily repeated very often, and at very short intervals.

Of course, these enormous copulative powers are not only *not* examples, but *contrasts* to what should obtain in the human being. As man has no real rutting season (which in animals appears to be a kind of periodic puberty), there is no occasion, and therefore no provision for the sudden or excessive employment of his reproductive organs, and consequently any such excesses will be fraught with much danger. The animal, moreover, is deficient in the intellectual qualities of man : propagation of his species appears to be about the most important of the objects of his existence. Man is formed for higher purposes than this. To devote the whole energy of his nature to sensual indulgence is literally to degrade himself to the level of an animal, and to impair or totally destroy those intellectual and moral capacities which distinguish him from the beast. Even in animals a limit is placed to sexual indulgence, and we find in some cases very curious physical provisions for attaining this end.

Among the preparations in the College of Surgeons' Museum may be seen the penis of the young tom-cat. It is described by Owen in the catalogue as " penis of a cat, showing the retroverted callous papillæ of the glans," and it is covered with spinous-looking elevations, which, in connection, must give the female much pain. They disappear in the old tom. The same conformation, or rather to a much greater extent, exists even in the guinea-pig. It is supposed that this rugous state of the male organ excites, if not anger, the greatest pain in the female.

Mr. Thompson, late Superintendent at the Zoological Gardens, corroborates the statement that in the feline race it is the female that makes the noise. He notices it as occurring constantly in leopards, tigers, lions, &c., and as presaging the conclusion of

not allow any horse in his establishment to mount more than twice a day. Two trials are generally advisable, as the first leap is often a failure. Country-travelling stallions are said to have stimulants given them, and to have as many as two hundred mounts in the season.

The bee is the example which at once suggests itself of one impregnation exhibiting its utmost limit of efficiency.

In the recent work of Siebold, translated by Dallas, entitled "On the True Parthenogenesis in Moths and Bees," a very interesting account is given of the act in the latter insects:

"It would appear that, whilst in the higher animals the male is the perfect and ruling creature—the bull keeps together, and, as it were, governs the herd of cattle, and the cock does the same by the hens—the reverse of this takes place in insects. In the wasps, hornets, humble bees, ants, and especially in the bees, the perfect female forms the central point, and holds the swarm together." (p. 40.) "Copulation never takes place in the hive. When the queen takes her wedding flight in fine warm weather, she makes her selection of a male bee (drone), and the act takes place in the air. It is very quickly completed, whereas other insects may remain for days united in copulation. When the queen returns to the hive after this single copulative act, the external orifice of the sexual apparatus, which was kept closed before the wedding flight, stands open, and the torn male copulative organs remain sticking in the vagina, and partly protrude from it. This eunuchism, Siebold says, not unfrequently occurs in other insects, as in the beetles. In the particular case examined by Siebold, the seminal receptacle (spermatheca), which is empty in all virgin female insects, was in this queen filled to overflowing with spermatozoids.

"In the copulation of the queen the ovary is not impregnated, but this vesicle, or seminal receptacle, is penetrated or filled by the male semen. By this, much—nay, all—of what was enigmatical is solved, especially how the queen can lay fertile eggs in the early spring, when there are no males in the hive. The supply of semen received during copulation is sufficient for her whole life. The copulation takes place once for all. The queen then never flies out again, except when the whole colony removes. When she has begun to lay, we may without scruple cut off her wings, she will still remain fertile until her death. But in her youth every queen must have flown out at least once, because the fertilization only takes place in the air; therefore no queen which has been lame in her wings from birth can ever be perfectly fertile. I say perfectly fertile, or capable of producing both sexes; for to lay drones' eggs, according to my experience, requires no fecundation at all." (p. 41.)

"After this single fecundation a queen bee can for a long time (four or five years) lay male or female eggs *at will;* for by filling her seminal receptacle with male semen she has acquired the power of producing female eggs; whilst before copulation, and with an empty seminal capsule, and therefore in the virgin state, she can only lay male eggs." (p. 53.)

The possibility of the semen thus lying in the spermatheca is a fact of great significance and importance, and illustrates the fact that seminal animalcules will live and thrive in the upper portion of the vagina long after they have been emitted from the testes.

Nature has, however, not only given the adult animal these instincts, but provides in a most wonderful way for their gratification.

SEXUAL ATTRACTION.—The devices, so to speak, which nature employs to bring the sexes together, are among the most interesting facts of zoology. No one can fail to notice the wonderful design evinced in bringing the sexes together by means of a phosphorescent light, as is the case with luminous insects. " The glowworm (*Lampyris noctiluca*) is an animal resembling a caterpillar ; its light proceeds from a pale-colored patch, that terminates the under side of the abdomen. It is, indeed, the perfect female of a winged beetle, from which it is altogether so different that nothing but actual observation could have inferred the fact of their being the different sexes of the same insect. The object of the light appears to be to attract the male, since it is most brilliant in the female, and in some species, if not all, is present only in the season when the sexes are destined to meet, and strikingly more vivid at the very moment when the meeting takes place. The torch which the wingless female, doomed to crawl upon the grass, lights up at the approach of night, is a beacon which unerringly guides the vagrant male to her 'lone illumined form,' however obscure the place of her abode."[1] The cause of this light is doubtless phosphorus, and we have reason to suppose that this is expended to a great extent in the act of copulation.

MARITAL DUTIES.—As I have advised continence, absolute and entire, for the young and the unmarried, so not the less urgently would I impress on the married the duty, for their own sakes, of *moderation* in sexual indulgence.

None, perhaps, but medical men can know at all (and they can know but a fraction of) the misery and suffering caused by ill-regulated desires and extravagant indulgences among married people. (See Marital Excesses, at page 148.)

Antiquity was sensible of the expediency of regulating to some

[1] Kirby and Spence, vol. ii. p. 420.

extent these indulgences. Many ordinances existed among ancient nations for the purpose, of which I give a few examples.

The following is a freely translated extract from the " Uxor Hebraica " of John Selden, lib. iii, cap. 6 (in his works, ed. 1646, vol. ii, pp. 717–720):

"They would have the conjugal debt paid regularly by the husband in proportion to the energy unused in his avocation. According to the Misna, a man was allowed one or two weeks' leave of absence on the score of a religious vow of abstinence. Law students were exempt. A weekly debt was forced upon artificers, but a daily one upon vigorous young husbands having no occupation. Donkey drivers (employed in transport of merchandise, &c.) were liable once a week ; camel-drivers (a calling entailing much labor and travelling) once in thirty days; sailors once (at any time) in six months. This is according to the Rabbi Eliezer."

Solon required three payments a month, without reference to the husband's avocations.

Mottery states in his " Travels," vol. i, p. 250, that the Turkish law obliges husbands to cohabit with their wives once a week, and that if they neglect to do so, the wife can lodge a complaint before a magistrate.

My own opinion is that, *taking hard-worked intellectual married men residing in London as the type*, sexual congress ought not to take place more frequently than once in seven or ten days; and when my opinion is asked by patients whose natural desires are strong, I advise those wishing to control their passions to indulge in intercourse twice on the same night. I have noticed that in many persons a single intercourse does not effectually empty the vasa deferentia, and that within the next twenty-four hours strong sexual feelings again arise; whereas, if sexual intercourse is repeated on the same night, the patient is able to so restrain his feelings that ten days or a fortnight may elapse without the recurrence of desire. The advantage of a second emission may be further considered with reference to statements on page 209, where I notice the probability that one vas deferens is only emptied at each emission. I believe the non-observance of some such rule as this is a very frequent cause of sterility in the female, as the spermatozoa are not fully formed.

The comments that have been made on these statements, as pub-

10

chapter entitled " Rules for Married Persons, or Matrimonial Chastity," he says :

" In their permissions and license, they must be sure to observe the order of nature and the ends of God. *He is an ill husband that uses his wife as a man treats a harlot*, having no other end but pleasure. Concerning which our best rule is, that although in this, as in eating and drinking, there is an appetite to be satisfied, which cannot be done without pleasing that desire, yet since that desire and satisfaction was intended by nature for other ends, they should never be separate from those ends, but always be joined with all or one of these ends, *with a desire of children, or to avoid fornication, or to lighten and ease the cares and sadnesses of household affairs, or to endear each other ;* but never with a purpose, either in act or desire, to separate the sensuality from these ends which hallow it.

" Married persons must keep such modesty and decency of treating each other that they never force themselves into high and violent lusts with arts and misbecoming devices ; always remembering that those mixtures are most innocent which are *most simple* and *most natural, most orderly* and *most safe*. It is the duty of matrimonial chastity to be restrained and temperate in the use of their lawful pleasures ; concerning which, although no universal rule can antecedently be given to all persons, any more than to all bodies one proportion of meat and drink, yet married persons are to estimate the degree of their license according to the following proportions.—1. That it be moderate, so as to consist with health. 2. That it be so ordered as not to be too expensive of time, that precious opportunity of working out our salvation. 3. That when duty is demanded, it be always paid (so far as in our powers and election) according to the foregoing measures. 4. That it be with a temperate affection, without violent transporting desires or too sensual applications. Concerning which a man is to make judgment by proportion to other actions and the severities of his religion, and the sentences of sober and wise persons, always remembering that marriage is a provision for supply of the natural necessities of the body, not for the artificial and procured appetites of the mind. And it is a sad truth that many married persons thinking that the floodgates of liberty are set wide open, without measures or restraints (so they sail in the channel), have felt the final rewards of intemperance and lust by their unlawful using of lawful permissions. Only let each of them be temperate, and both of them be modest. Socrates was wont to say that those women to whom nature hath not been indulgent in good features and colors should make it up themselves with excellent manners, and those who were beautiful and comely should be careful that so fair a body be not polluted with unhandsome usages. To which Plutarch adds, that a wife, if she be unhandsome, should consider how extremely ugly she should be if she wanted modesty ; but if she be handsome, let her think how gracious that beauty would be if she superadds chastity." (P. 70, Bell and Daldy edition, 1857.)

Let me add the advice of a still older writer, who, on these subjects, amid much quaintness has many most sound and excellent remarks—Chaucer.

"An for that many a man," he says, "weeneth he may not sinne for no lecherousness that he doth with his wife, certes that opinion is false; God wot a man may slay himself with his own knife, and make himself drunk with his own tun. Man should love his wife by discretion—patiently and temperately. . . . .

" Then shall man understand that for three things a man and his wife may fleshly assemble (come together). The first is in intent of engendure of children to the service of God—for certes that is the cause final of matrimony, for neither of them has power of his own body. The second cause is to yield every of them his debt unto other of his body. The third is to eschew lechery and villany. The fourth forsooth is deadly sin. . . . . Understand that if they assemble only for amorous love, and for none of the foresaid causes, but for to accomplish that burning delight, they reck never how oft, soothly, it is deadly sin; and yet, with sorrow, some folk will more pain them for to do, than to their appetite sufficeth." ("Chaucer's Canterbury Tales," " The Parson's Tale.")

PART II.

DISORDERS IN THE ADULT.

CHAPT. I.—MARITAL EXCESSES.

IT is a common notion among the public, and even among professional men, that the word *excess* chiefly applies to *illicit* sexual connection. Of course, whether extravagant in degree or not, all such connection is, from one point of view, *an excess*. But any warning against sexual dangers would be very incomplete if it did not extend to the excesses too often committed by married persons in ignorance of their ill effects. Too frequent emissions of the life-giving fluid, and too frequent sexual excitement of the nervous system are, as we have seen, in themselves most destructive. The result is the same within the marriage bond as without it. The married man who thinks that, because he is a married man, he can commit no excess, however often the act of sexual congress is repeated, will suffer as certainly and as seriously as the unmarried debauchee who acts on the same principle in his indulgences—perhaps more certainly, from his very ignorance, and from his not taking those precautions and following those rules which a career of vice is apt to teach the sensualist. Many a man has, until his marriage, lived a most continent life; so has his wife. As soon as they are wedded, intercourse is indulged in night after night; neither party having any idea that these repeated sexual acts are excesses which the system of neither can bear, and which to the man, at least, is absolute ruin. The practice is continued till health is impaired, sometimes permanently; and when a patient is at last obliged to seek medical advice, he is thunderstruck at learning that his sufferings arise from excesses unwittingly committed. Married people often appear to think that connection may be repeated just as regularly and almost as often as' their meals. Till they are told of the danger the idea never enters their heads that they have been guilty of great and almost criminal excess; nor is this to be wondered at, since the possibility of such a cause of disease is seldom hinted at by the medical man they consult.

Some years ago a young man called on me, complaining that he was unequal to sexual congress, and was suffering from spermatorrhœa, the result, he said, of self-abuse. He was cauterized, and I lost sight of him until March, 1856, when he returned, complaining that he was scarcely able to move alone. His mind had become enfeebled, there was great pain in the back, and he wished me to repeat the operation.

On cross-examining the patient, I found that after the previous cauterization he had recovered his powers, and, having subsequently married, had been in the habit of indulging in connection (ever since I had seen him, two years previously) three times a week, without any idea that he was committing an excess, or that his present weakness could depend upon this cause. The above is far from being an isolated instance of men who, having been reduced by former excesses, still imagine themselves equal to any excitement, and when their powers are recruited, to any expenditure of vital force. Some go so far as to believe that indulgence may increase these powers, just as gymnastic exer-

and about the same time his sexual powers gradually became impaired. The real object, he avowed, which he had in coming to me was to obtain some stimulus to increase his sexual powers, rather than to gain relief for the nervousness and debility under which he was laboring. Indeed, at his request, the efforts of the country practitioner had been made in the former direction. Instead of giving remedies to excite, I told him that his convalescence must depend upon moderate indulgence, and allowing the system to rally, and treated him accordingly.

The lengths to which some married people carry excesses is perfectly astonishing. I lately saw a married medical man who told me that for the last fourteen years, he believed, he had *never* allowed a night to pass without having had connection, and it was only lately, on reading my book, that he had attributed his present ailments to marital excesses. The contrast between such a case as this, where an individual for fourteen years has resisted this drain on the system, and that of a man who is, as many are, prostrated for twenty-four hours by one nocturnal emission, is most striking. This great disparity is further discussed at page 231. All experience, however, shows that, whatever may be the condition of the nervous system, as regards sexual indulgences, excesses sooner or later tell upon any frame, and can never be indulged in with impunity. I believe too frequent sexual relations to be much more common than is generally supposed, and that they are hardly yet sufficiently appreciated by the profession as very fruitful causes of ill health.

I will give one more instance. A medical man called on me, saying he found himself suffering from spermatorrhœa. There were general debility, inaptitude to work, and disinclination for sexual intercourse; in fact he thought he was losing his senses and the sight of one eye was affected. The only way in which he lost semen was, as he thought, by slight occasional oozing from the penis. I asked him at once if he had ever committed excesses. As a boy, he acknowledged having abused himself, but he married seven years previously to his visit to me, being then a hearty, healthy man, and it was only lately that he had been complaining. In answer to my further inquiry, he stated that since his marriage he had had connection two or three times a week, and often more than once a night. This one fact, I was obliged to tell him, sufficiently accounted for all his troubles. The symptoms he complained of were similar to those we find in boys who abuse themselves. It is true that it may take years to reduce some strong, healthy men, just as it may be a long time before some boys are prejudicially influenced, but the ill effects of excesses are sooner or later sure to follow.

Since my attention has been particularly called to this class of ailments, I feel confident that many of the forms of indigestion, general ill health, hypochondriasis, &c., so often met with in adults, depend upon sexual excesses. The directors of hydropathic establishments must probably hold some such opinions, or they would not have thought it expedient to separate married patients when they are undergoing the water treatment. That this cause of illness is not more widely acknowledged and acted on, arises from the natural delicacy which medical men must feel in putting such questions to their patients as are necessary to elicit the facts.

I have often been surprised at the immediate and manifest benefit produced in these cases by enjoining moderate indulgence or complete *abstinence*, together with the simple treatment hereafter detailed under the head of Spermatorrhœa, when other remedies have entirely failed.

It may very naturally be asked what is meant by an *excess* in sexual indulgence. The simple reply is—the same as in any other indulgence. An excess is what injures health. I have at page 145 stated that, according to my experience, few hardworking intellectual married men should indulge in connection *oftener* than once in seven or perhaps ten days. This, however, is only a guide for strong, healthy men. Generally, I should say that an individual may consider he has committed an *excess*, when coitus is succeeded by languor, depression of spirits, and malaise. This is the safest definition! Such results should not happen if the male is in good health and indulges his sexual desires moderately.

No invariable law can be laid down in a case where so much

must depend upon temperament, age, climate, and other circumstances, as well as the health and strength of both parties. I maintain that in highly civilized communities the continuance of a high degree of bodily and mental vigor is inconsistent with more than a *very moderate* indulgence in sexual intercourse. The still higher principle also holds good that man was not created only to indulge his sexual appetites, and that he should subordinate them to his other duties.

It is not the body alone which suffers from excesses committed in married life. Experience every day convinces me that much of the languor of mind, confusion of ideas, and inability to control the thoughts of which some married men complain, arises from this cause. These ill effects are noticed not unfrequently in patients who have married late in life, and still more often in persons who have married a second time after having been widowers for some years.

The ill effects of marital excesses are not confined to offending parties. No doubt can exist that many of the obscure cases of sickly children born of apparently healthy parents arise from this cause, and this is borne out by investigations among animals.

M. Goddard has related some interesting experiments made at the Haras of Poitou on the liquid ejaculated by stallions in their different jumps on the same day. He has established that the semen, which was tolerably thick and very opaline, of an amber color in the first jump, became more and more clear, and less and less thick, so that after the fourth jump the liquid was absolutely like water, and scarcely contained any animalcules. It was thus easy by the eye alone to distinguish the semen ejaculated by the same animal at different times of the day. According to the same observer, the semen of the first jump of a morning would possess alone certain fecundating properties, and in a covering establishment it would be advantageous to allow the same animal only one jump a day, one jump every second day would be even preferable. By acting in this way the owner would obtain a better result than by obliging stallions to jump four or five time in the twenty-four hours.—"*Traité de Physiologie Longet*," p. 779.

1. Sexual Indifference or Temporary Absence of Desire.

We have treated in preceding pages of the evil of any excess in the indulgence of the sex-passions; we now come to the consideration of at least as great an evil, the partial or total absence of the passion itself.

Sexual Indifference among Single Men.—This condition may arise from a variety of *causes.* We find, for instance, that some men reach adult age without having experienced any sexual desire at all. That complete sexual quiescence which we have noticed as being the proper condition of childhood continues in cases such as we are describing, during the period of youth, and even into adult age.

In some it is only at an unusually late period that the natural sexual desire commences; this delay in the development of the reproductive powers gives rise to a variety of surmises, but curiously enough the patient himself is the last person alarmed at the delay in the appearance of sexual feeling, and it is often only accidentally that a medical man is consulted about it at all.

Prognosis.—It does not necessarily follow in such cases that the existing impotence is anything but temporary. In the case described above there may be a late development of the organs. Instead of the young man being precocious, circumstances may simply have delayed the structural and functional maturing of the testes, which, under proper treatment, may still be perfected.

Treatment.—It must naturally be inferred that little can be done in the alleviation of this form of the complaint, except waiting patiently the results of puberty, and by every means in our power invigorating the patient's constitution. Marriage, of course, must not be thought of so long as the sexual powers are undeveloped.

There is another and very different cause which often produces a kind of temporary impotence, that creates much unnecessary anxiety. The student, who previously has experienced all the sexual desires common to his age, all at once, during any strenuous and long-continued mental exertion while he is absorbed in his studies, finds all sexual feelings annihilated. Men who are

these that furnish funds for the advertising firms who fill the pages of some of our country and London journals with their trashy advertisements. These harpies fatten on the ignorances and prejudices of such patients, humor their fears, increasing and exaggerating the supposed consequences, and only turn them adrift when they have emptied their pockets. If, however, a sympathetic and competent medical man be consulted, he can conscientiously inform them, that a youth who first falls in love is often beset by these alarms, which I have classed under the symptoms of false impotence, and that a little sympathy on the part of the surgeon, with some confidence on the part of the patient, and the treatment recommended at page 77, will suffice to effect a cure, and enable him to marry, when all his alarms will cease by the proof that his sexual powers have been unimpaired, and that without care on his part, the patient may rather be in danger of giving way to the marital excesses alluded to at page 148.

It should be recollected that there are other causes producing indifference to the opposite sex and deficiency in manly vigor. The most common of such causes is the wretched habit of masturbation, of which we have already treated. A youth who masturbates himself and continues the practice as he grows up to manhood, may evince, even after he has arrived at the marriageable age, no disposition towards the other sex. Only his own solitary pleasure can give him any gratification; as far as women are concerned, he is virtually impotent. Lallemand gives the following perhaps rather too[1] graphic account of such a person's

---

[1] I think I ought at once to state that, although we are very much indebted to this distinguished Professor for having written a most valuable treatise on seminal losses, yet the reader must not be led away with the idea that every young man who has been a victim to the vice would suffer as described in this paragraph, or that I would say, "ex uno disce omnes." We must consider these as symptoms in sufferers who have carried the vice to its utmost limits; and the illustrations are not given as ordinary tpyical cases, but as the most strongly marked. I have cited Lallemand for this reason, but I may add, that in my extensive experience I have seldom met with such cases as these, and when I have done so it has usually been in persons who, from having had no one to consult or sympathize with them, have exaggerated their miseries by morbidly dwelling upon them.

adopted this as the easiest and least embarrassing mode of telling an otherwise long and painful story.

I remain, my dear Sir, yours, &c.

W. ACTON, Esq.

The writer was a tall, gentlemanly young man. He assured me that he masturbated himself in sleep in spite of all his efforts, and that it particularly occurred after taking wine. He did not find the desire irresistible during his waking moments, except after he had failed in attempting intercourse with women, when, in a kind of despair, he generally yielded to the old temptation. To avoid the practice during sleep, he had sometimes been compelled to tie his wrists together by a cord that passed round his neck, so as to prevent himself from touching the penis. I have known several such cases, where patients who wished to cure themselves of the habit of masturbation have, against their feelings, sought the society of women, have attempted connection in vain, and then have come to me, ashamed of their failure, disgusted with themselves for the vice, and apparently almost ready to commit suicide from despair and misery. Others have confessed to me that, though sexual intercourse has been attended with difficulty, still the act was accomplished, but that it was attended with no pleasure. As their own self-pollution could still afford them gratification, they acknowledged that they fell back to their old vice, of which they were all the time thoroughly ashamed.

This strange phenomenon, of self-abuse affording greater gratification than intercourse with the other sex, the idea of whom, after all, creates the excitement, is more common than is generally supposed, and more in accordance with what we should expect than at first sight appears. The confirmed masturbator, as Rousseau has described, has to picture in his imagination all the female charms that can exist, so as to be able to rouse his flagging sexual desires. But when he attempts for the first time, or at long intervals, to accomplish sexual intercourse, he finds much difficulty and very little pleasure. He is probably naturally timid, he dreads the exposure of his infirmities, he fears contamination, and is, on the whole, thoroughly ill at ease. His ignorance, his conscience, the very novelty of his position, and the dread of consequences, tend, for the time, to paralyze his sexual desires.

Another explanation, also to some extent true, is that the nervous system, and particularly the sympathetic system, has been so often and repeatedly excited that it will only respond to the particular kind of stimulus to which it has become accustomed, and is proof against all others.

If, then, it be true that among single men we meet with cases of well-marked sexual indifference, lasting only for a short time, and giving rise to very little annoyance to the patient, so it is no less true that we more frequently than otherwise meet with cases where the assumed impotence exists only in the imagination of the married man, causing one of the most painful forms of monomania that it is the duty of the consulting surgeon to treat. These cases require more attention than has hitherto been given to them, and I shall now proceed to give my readers an account of the affection which they will often meet with in private practice.

SEXUAL INDIFFERENCE AMONG MARRIED MEN, as a temporary affection, is another cause of anxiety, which in some persons produces the greatest alarm.

Causes.—Men who gain their bread by the sweat of their brows, or the exhausting labor of their brains, should be made aware that they cannot expect to be always ready to perform the sexual act. During certain periods, when occupied with other matters, man's thoughts dwell but little on sexual subjects, and no disposition exists to indulge anything but the favorite or absorbing pursuit, mental or physical as the case may be. After a lapse of time, different in various individuals, sexual thoughts recur, and the man who yesterday was so indifferent to sexual feelings, as practically to be temporarily impotent, now becomes ardent and sexually disposed, remaining so until the necessary and in fact, healthy lethargy of the organs follows the performance of the act.

This quiescent condition is much more persistent in some

married men than in others. There are persons (married as well as single) who only at very infrequent intervals feel any disposition for sexual intercourse, just as there are others who never feel any such desire at all. Again, there are *lethargic* men, who, unless roused, will hardly do anything. It requires an effort in some men to eat. There is in some of these cases undoubtedly great sexual debility. Again, the habitual drinker cares little for sexual enjoyments.. I am quite certain that some excessive smokers, if very young, never acquire, and if older, rapidly lose any keen desire for connection. The pleasures of the table so monopolize many a man's thoughts that he is indifferent to all other indulgences. In all the above cases the sexual feelings occupy a secondary position, and never attain, or even approach, that tyrannous mastery from which the thorough voluptuary suffers. It is in these advanced stages of this condition, often difficult to say whether the sexual organization was originally weak, whether the other tastes have overpowered the sexual appetite, or whether the individual has not early in life abused his generative faculty.

Among the married we sometimes find men taking a dislike or even a disgust to their wives, and, as a consequence, there is an entire want of desire. A first failure will sometimes so annihilate men's sexual appetite that they are never able or anxious to attempt connection a second time. In many cases this arises from wounded *amour propre*, as they succeed with other women. Early excesses in married life will, in a certain number of cases, occasionally produce a temporary impotency later in life. Want of sympathy or want of sexual feeling on the woman's part, again, is not an unfrequent cause of apathy, indifference, or frigidity on the part of the husband. Lastly, there are cases of amiable men who carry their consideration for the women they love to such an extent as to render themselves practically impotent for very dread of inflicting pain. A singularly agreeable and gentlemanly, but very mild looking man, once called on me, saying that he had been lately married, and had not succeeded in performing his marital duties. I treated him in the usual way and he got better, but still the act was not satisfactorily

11

strong that they surpass those of men, and shock public feeling by their consequences. I admit, of course, the existence of sexual excitement terminating even in nymphomania,[1] a form of insanity that those accustomed to visit lunatic asylums must be fully conversant with; but, with these sad exceptions, there can be no doubt that sexual feeling in the female is in the majority of cases in abeyance, and that it requires positive and considerable excitement to be roused at all: and even if roused (which in many instances it never can be) it is very moderate compared with that of the male. Many persons, and particularly young men, form their ideas of women's sensuous feelings from what they notice early in life among loose or, at least, low and vulgar women. There is always a certain number of females who, though not ostensibly in the ranks of prostitutes, make a kind of trade of a pretty face. They are fond of admiration, they like to attract the attention of those immediately above them. Any susceptible boy is easily led to believe, whether he is altogether overcome by the syren or not, that she, and therefore all women, must have at least as strong passions as himself. Such women, however, give a very false idea of the condition of female sexual feeling in general. Association with the loose women of the London streets in casinos and other immoral haunts (who, if they have not sexual feeling, counterfeit it so well that the novice does not suspect but that it is genuine), seems to corroborate such an impression, and as I have stated above, it is from these erroneous notions that so many unmarried men think that the marital duties they will have to undertake are beyond their exhausted strength, and from this reason dread and avoid marriage.

[1] I shall probably have no other opportunity of noticing that, as excision of the clitoris has been recommended for the cure of this complaint, Köbelt thinks that it would not be necessary to remove the whole of the clitoris in nymphomania, the same results (that is destruction of veneral desire) would follow if the glans clitoridis had been alone removed, as it is now considered that it is in the glands alone in which the sensitive nerves expand. This view I do not agree with, as I have already stated with regard to the analogous structure of the penis, p. 134. I am fully convinced that in many women there is no special sexual sensation in the clitoris, and I am positive that the special sensibility dependent on the erectile tissue exists in several portions of the vaginal canal.

and that even then there was some doubt as to the completion of the act. He brought his wife with him, as she was, he said, desirous of having some conversation with me.

I found the lady a refined but highly sensitive person. Speaking with a freedom equally removed from assurance, or *mauvaise honte*, she told me she thought it her duty to consult me. She neither blushed nor faltered in telling her story, and I regret that my words must fail to convey the delicacy with which her avowal was made.

Her husband and herself, she said, had been acquainted from childhood, had grown up together, became mutually attached, and married. She had reason to consider him debilitated, but— as she was fully convinced—from no indiscreet acts on his part. She believed it was his natural condition. She was dotingly attached to him, and would not have determined to consult me, but that she wished for his sake, to have a family, as it would, she hoped, conduce to their mutual happiness. She assured me that she felt no sexual passions whatever ; that if she was capable of them they were dormant. Her passion for her husband was of a Platonic kind, and far from wishing to stimulate his frigid feelings, she doubted whether it would be right or not. She loved him as he was, and would not desire him to be otherwise except for the hope of having a family.

I believe this lady is a perfect ideal of an English wife and mother, kind, considerate, self-sacrificing, and sensible, so pure-hearted as to be utterly ignorant of and averse to any sensual indulgence, but so unselfishly attached to the man she loves, as to be willing to give up her own wishes and feelings for his sake.

In strong contrast to the unselfish sacrifices such married women make of their feelings in allowing cohabitation, stand out others, who, either from ignorance or utter want of sympathy, although they are model wives in every other respect, not only evince no sexual feeling, but, on the contrary, scruple not to declare their aversion to the least manifestation of it. Doubtless this may, and often does, depend upon disease, and if so, the sooner the suffering female is treated the better. Much more frequently, however, it depends upon apathy, selfish indifference to please, or unwillingness to overcome a natural repugnance for cohabitation.

Other mental conditions may influence the female. Thus, the High Church enthusiast may consider it her strictly religious duty to be separated from her husband during the forty days of Lent; and at page 263 I shall give an instance of a wife refusing to cohabit with her husband because she would not again become a mother. I was lately in conversation with a lady who maintains woman's rights to such an extent that she denied the husband any voice in the matter, whether or not cohabitation should take place. She maintained, most strenuously, that as the woman bears the consequences—has all the discomfort of being nine months in the family-way, and thus is obliged to give up her amusements and many of her social relations—considering too that she suffers all the pains and risks of childbirth—a married woman has a perfect right to refuse to cohabit with her husband. I ventured to inform this strong-minded female that such conduct on her part might be, in a medical point of view, highly detrimental to the health of the husband, particularly if he happened to be strongly sexually disposed. She refused to admit the validity of my argument, and replied that such a man, unable to control his feelings, ought to have married a street-walker, not an intellectually disposed person, who could not and ought not to be obliged to devote her time to duties only compatible with the position of a female drudge or wet-nurse.

I am not prepared to say how far Lord Penzance would receive such evidence in the case of a man seeking a divorce, and I am not aware that counsel has as yet urged such conduct on the part of the female in extenuation of immorality on the part of the husband. Of one thing I am quite certain that many times in the course of the year I am consulted by conscientious married men, who complain, and I think with reason, that they are debarred from the privileges of marriage, and that their sexual sufferings are great in consequence of being mated to women who think and act as in the above cited instances. I regret to add that medical skill can be of little avail here. The more conscientious the husband and the stronger his sexual feelings, the more distressing are the sufferings he is doomed to undergo, ultimately too often ending in impotence.

Perversion of Sexual Feeling.—Where, in addition to the indisposition to cohabitation which many modest women feel, we find a persistent aversion to it, so strong as to be invincible by entreaty or by any amount of kindness on the husband's part, a very painful suspicion may sometimes arise as to the origin of so unconquerable a frigidity.

The following is a case in which these suspicions seemed to be justified by the facts:—A gentleman came to ask my opinion on the cause of want of sexual feeling in his wife. He told me he had been married four years. His wife was about his own age (twenty-seven), and had had four children, but she evinced no sexual feeling, although a lively, healthy lady, living in the country. I suggested several causes, when he at last asked me if it was possible that a woman might lose sexual feeling from the same cause as men. "I have read your former edition, Mr. Acton," said he, "and though you only allude to the subject incidentally, yet from what I have learned since my marriage, I am led to think that my wife's want of sexual feeling may arise, if you can affirm to me that such a thing is possible, from self-abuse. She has confessed to me that at a boarding-school, in perfect ignorance of any injurious effects, she early acquired the habit. This practice still gives her gratification; not so connection, which she views with positive aversion, although it gives her no pain." I told him that medical men who are consulted about female complaints, have not unfrequently observed cases like that of his wife. It appears that, at last, nothing but the morbid excitement produced by the baneful practice can give any sexual gratification, and that the natural stimulus fails to cause any pleasure whatever. A similar phenomenon occurs in men, and this state is seldom got the better of as long as self-abuse is practised. I feared, therefore, that his surmises were correct, and that the lady practised self-abuse more frequently than she was willing to admit. So ruinous is the practice of solitary vice, both in the one and other sex, so difficult is it to give it up, that I fear it may be carried on even in married life, where

no excuse can be devised, and may actually come to be preferred
to the natural excitement. Venereal excesses engender satiety
just as certainly as any other indulgences, and satiety is followed
by indifference and disgust. If the unnatural excesses of masturbation take place early in life, before the subjects who commit
them have arrived at maturity, it is not surprising that we meet
with women whose sexual feelings, if they ever existed, become
prematurely worn out. Doubtless sexual feeling differs largely
in different women; and although it is not my object to treat
otherwise than incidentally of the sexual economy in women, yet
I may here say that the causes which in early life induces abnormal sexual excitement in boys operate in a similar manner on
girls. This tendency may be checked in girls, as in boys, by
careful moral education in early life. But no doubt can exist
that hereditary predisposition has much to do with this, independently of education and early associations. It is publicly
maintained by some credible persons that there are well-known
families, for instance, in which chastity is not a characteristic
feature among the females. We offer, I hope, no apology for
light conduct when we admit that there are some *few* women who,
like men, in consequence of hereditary predisposition or ill-
directed moral education, find it difficult to restrain their passions, while their more fortunate sisters have never been tempted,
and have, therefore, never fallen. This, however, does not alter
the fact which I would venture again to impress on the reader,
that, in general, women do *not* feel any great sexual tendencies.
The unfortunately large numbers whose lives would seem to
prove the contrary are to be otherwise accounted for. Vanity,
giddiness, greediness, love of dress, distress, or hunger, make
women prostitutes, but do not induce female profligacy so largely
as has been supposed.[1]

II. True Impotence.

1st Stage. Permanent Absence of Desire.—So unusual
a phenomenon as an entire absence of sexual desires, alluded to

[1] See Author's work on "Prostitution," 2d edition, p. 167.

at p. 170, must always be rather an alarming and suspicious circumstance. Unfortunately in the majority of such cases the medical man is seldom consulted at an early period, as neither the patient nor his friends are aware that there is anything unusual in his condition until it is accidentally discovered. The surgeon appealed to will usually find that the individual is fat, without hair on his face, or even down on the pubes, the testes and penis are small, almost rudimentary, like those of a young child,[1] there is no sexual desire, and the voice is often weak and almost falsetto in quality ; in fact, the condition is much the same as that of the castrated individual or eunuch.[2]

In such a case it is clear that an imperfect development of the testes has resulted in a state of eunuchism, accompanied by many of the peculiarities which, both in animals and in human beings, follow on castration.

This partially undeveloped state of the reproductive system usually indicates itself, among other signs, by a marked indifference to manly sports and exercises, and a visible deficiency in virile attributes generally.

If, however, on examination, it should appear that the testes,

---

[1] Dr. Davy has given the following post-mortem appearances in a patient who showed (according to the account given by his comrades) an aversion to the sex. "There was little hair on pubes or chin, the *partes naturales* were all small, the larynx was small, the skin delicate. A very minute portion of fluid only could be procured from the vasa deferentia, which under the microscope exhibited numerous small particles and a few larger globules, but no spermatic animalcules. The fluid of the *vesiculæ* was also small in quantity and destitute of animalcules ; it was of a light-brownish hue, slightly opaque, containing some globules, and did not change the color of turmeric or of litmus paper. The fluid from their fundus was most gelatinous and appeared to consist chiefly of mucus. The *vesiculæ seminales* in this instance and their contents resembled those of such castrated animals as I have hitherto examined." ("Edinburgh Medical and Surgical Journal," vol. L, p. 7.)

[2] Pope Clement XIV, in the eighteenth century, abolished castration of youths, which was then practised in Italy for the purpose of retaining the soprano voice. It is well known that the castrated preserve the shrill voice (*voix aigue*) of infancy, at the same time that the chest becomes fully developed, thus giving volume to the voice. Women were not allowed to sing in the cathedral or church services, hence this horrid mutilation, as it qualified the victim to sing soprano parts.

instead of being merely small, are little more than rudimentary organs; if they are apparently mere nodules; if this change of structure has followed an early attack of mumps or some inflammatory affection of the testes, or an accident which has injured them early in life, the case must, I fear, be considered as a hopeless one, and the patient should be treated as permanently impotent. Terrible as this doom may seem, it is singular to notice how indifferent such persons appear to their deficiency. They do not know the value of what they never possessed and never will possess, and they pass through life contented men, evincing neither aversion to, or liking for the opposite sex.

It may be some satisfaction for nervous patients who may read these pages to be reminded that the really impotent men are, as a rule, thus indifferent to their symptoms; and I may lay it down as a general rule that a man who is very timid about the existence of impotence is not likely to be impotent at all, but only fears he may become so.

I. ABSENCE OR DEFICIENCY OF POWER.—INABILITY TO CONSUMMATE MARRIAGE.

"True impotence," says Lallemand, "consists in want of power in connection, not once, but habitually; not only with courtesans, but with those whom we most love; not under unfavorable circumstances, but during long periods of time, say, five, fifteen, or twenty years, when married to lovely and handsome women, whose devotion to their husbands has never been questioned." (Vol. ii, p. 242.)

That this lamentable state of things truly exists there can be no doubt, and in London those whose attention is devoted to diseases of the reproductive organs, occasionally meet with cases in which there appears to be complete annihilation of all the sexual feelings and actions, and in which the man is reduced to what Roubaud describes as *generative syncope*. Such instances, however, are rare. Usually it happens, at least in England, that the functional diseases requiring treatment consist in the absence of only one or more of the conditions necessary for coition. In the east, I am told, the Levantines are often perfectly impotent before they arrive at the age of thirty. If report speaks correctly, Hien Fung, the late Emperor of China, was in this condition.

The forms that impotence assumes are various, though the result is the same in all cases, viz., inability to perform the sexual act. Thus a man may be utterly impotent whether he has or has not erection attendant on desire. Again, there may be only a partial erection, lasting an insufficient length of time for penetration; or the erection may be so weak, or the emission so quick, as practically to render the man impotent; or a man may be impotent from emission not taking place at all; or emission may not occur until some time after connection has been attempted.

Causes.—I fear we must come to the conclusion that when there *is* desire, and merely a want of power, this state of things arises from abuse of the generative organs, aggravated in most instances by alarm, a guilty conscience, fear of not succeeding, habits of intemperance, or too free use of tobacco, from timidity, or from too frequent excitement without gratification.

The exact way in which these causes produce the effects of impotence is not certainly known, but it is most probably by occasioning lesions of the nervous system, and more especially of that portion which is under the influence of the sympathetic nerve or excito-motory system.

Non-descent of the Testes is a cause of impotence in some men, and it appears almost invariably to be attended by sterility. I do not pretend to say that every man who has an undescended testicle must necessarily be altogether impotent; a few cases are recorded of men whose testes had never descended into the scrotum having had families; but I have met with several instances, one of which I shall presently describe, where, I believe, impotence arose entirely from this cause. It is true that in the elephant, and some other animals, in the cetacea, in birds and reptiles, the testes are constantly found in the abdomen, side by side with the kidneys, lungs, &c. These facts point to the possibility that if the adult's testes are truly in the abdomen, they

and his conclusion was that in the Cryptorchis no seminal animalcules are ever found in the secretion, although the ejaculated fluid has been frequently examined. He concludes that "men both of whose testicles are arrested in their evolution are sterile, but not impotent; that those who have for their generative apparatus only vasa deferentia are sterile, and nearly incapable of sexual intercourse."—*Comptes rendus des séances de la Société de Biologie*, tome iii, série 2, 1856, p. 315.

My own experience in practice certainly is, that men with undescended testes have no family. I was consulted by a gentleman in 1861, in consequence of his wife having no children. My patient told me he had been married some years, and the lady presented all the external attributes of a person likely to have a large family, and I was aware that she had consulted a celebrated physician, at whose suggestion the husband had come to me. There was no suspicion on my part at the time that the testes were absent, or even imperfectly developed. However, on examination, it was impossible to detect any testicles in the scrotum, and pressure in the groin did not give the patient any peculiar pain. There was, nevertheless, abundant evidence that the testes existed, although they had not descended. In no other respect did the patient differ from other men, and he assured me that the sexual feeling was natural, and that he had connection once or twice a week, the emission being as abundant as he supposed it would be in other men. I must, notwithstanding, say that, as far as my personal observations go, I look with great suspicion on the procreative powers of any person with undescended testes.

Among other causes of impotence, or rather sterility, I may mention the influence of—

Hernia and Trusses.—Since the fourth edition of this book was published, I have paid considerable attention to this subject, and I think I may now state confidently that trusses may and often do most seriously interfere with the reproductive powers, and in a way that truss makers might readily obviate by adopting some improved construction. The object of mechanicians being solely to keep the hernia in place, the penis or testes are often so carelessly thrust aside or pressed upon, that their functions are seriously interfered with.

When a case of the kind comes under my care, and the patient complains of want of sexual power, I always examine how the truss presses. If I see any reason to suppose that it can by any possibility be the cause of the symptoms, I attempt in the first place by diet and abstinence from certain articles to cause absorption of fat in the mesentery and amentum; this being done, I attempt, but with great caution, to reduce the size of the truss. It is singular how often this can be effected with safety; I find that not only are the sexual powers often recovered when the pressure is thus relieved, but that the penis, when it is no longer thrust aside, regains its natural size where that has diminished.

I strongly object to strings crossing the abdomen, inasmuch as I think the procreative powers may very probably be interfered with when a double truss is worn; and in cases such as I speak of, where the impotence is the most marked feature, it becomes a serious question whether its use should be continued, particularly when, as in some instances, it has merely been sanctioned as a precautionary measure. I need not say, however, that if a truss on one side can be altogether dispensed with, the partial recovery of the reproductive powers will be more likely to be effected. I believe, moreover, that in many cases, great relief can be obtained by judicious alterations in the shape, size, and point of pressure, and in the method of attachment of the truss.

Varicocele, or enlargement of the veins of the chord, is another affection which, in its severer forms, if it does not *produce* impotence, at least aggravates it. Whenever a patient comes to me with this affection, I at once order a suspensory bandage, or what I prefer, a *varicocele ring,* an instrument formed of soft pliable metal, covered with wash leather. These are made of different sizes, and can be procured at Furgusson's, surgical instrument maker, Giltspur Street, City; or of Bell's or Corbyn's, Oxford Street. These rings, in the majority of cases, answer the purpose admirably, but when the scrotum is very thin or deficient in cellular tissue, they are liable to slip off. This may be obviated by tying a piece of thin twine to the ring, the other end of it being attached to the button of the drawers. The ring should be taken off at night, and only put on after the sponging-bath—it should be worn for some months.

Before leaving this branch of our subject, I shall remind the reader that all the practical results of impotence can be, and constantly are, produced by the mechanical effect of a—

Stricture of the urethra, by preventing the emission of semen. The description of this form of disease of the reproductive organs is not within the scope of the present treatise. For further information upon it I may refer to my larger work on the "Urinary and Generative Organs," page 81.

Impregnation is, of course, rendered almost impossible by a serious stricture, as the semen, instead of being at once ejaculated, can only dribble away afterwards when all erection has disappeared. The act of connection, moreover, is often painful, the pain being generally felt during the ejaculatory act. This form of impotence is amenable to treatment, such as dilatation and other proper measures for removing the stricture.

Impotence arising from a similar cause is observed in sheep. The high-fed and high-bred rams, from which the best breeds are obtained, become subject to a kind of stricture arising from the deposit of calcareous matter in the urethra. The peculiar conformation of the organ in sheep conduces to this result.[1]

---

[1] The glans penis of the ram consists of an oval and wrinkled swelling, divided horizontally at the end, looking like the head of a snake. From this glans projects a long, thin appendix, of a consistent character. This appendix, which shepherds call "the worm," tapers to a point, and the canal passing through it is very small. A ram is sometimes observed to be very uneasy and apparently to be less and less able to micturate. On examination, the vermiform appendage is found distended and stiffened from an accumulation of calcareous matter within the urethral canal. This in some instances can be removed by slightly pressing and rolling the appendix between the fingers, which will at once relieve the strangury, and save the animal, but frequently either the ram has to be killed or part of "the worm" be removed. If sufficient is left the ram may still be able to breed. And even if complete connection is impossible, breeders still use these mutilated animals, called "teazers," to excite the ewes, and so spare the valuable tups some fatigue.

That impotence then frequently depends upon the male becoming too fat may be considered as an established fact. There is every reason to believe that the same cause occasionally induces sterility in females.

I was lately in conversation with a gentleman, a large farmer in Suffolk. He told me that he is often disappointed when he wishes to breed from cart-mares. This year, out of his own working stock of twenty-eight horses, eleven mares did not *stand*, greatly to his disappointment and loss, as a yearling colt is worth twenty pounds, and the mare ceases work only during one month before and during one month after parturition. This sterility he attributes to the high condition his cattle are kept in by the carters, who, proud of their teams, do not care to see them in foal. To obviate it, fresh stallions have been purchased, and with as little success, sterility still prevailing. Amongst these eleven mares there were young as well as old ones, but none of them proved in foal.

The treatment of cases of Corpulence has within the last few years excited considerable attention, no doubt through the pamphlet of Mr. Banting, who, however, is indebted to Mr. Harvey, a member of our profession, for the plan he recommends. I have from the first strongly recommended the chief features of the system as beneficial for the general health, especially in the case of persons of a corpulent tendency. No doubt can exist that abstinence from, or extreme moderation in, fat, butter, milk, cream, bread, potatoes, sugar, and beer, will in one week considerably diminish the weight, and in fat persons remove many uncomfortable sensations. When a patient is over stout the weight may be fairly and safely reduced one or two pounds weekly. I have often found such treatment assist the recovery of sexual power in persons in whom it has been failing. This plan has been proved to work equally well with animals, and I have heard of several instances of over-fat bulls that had become impotent, recovering their procreative powers after being sent to work on the farm upon less food.

Abnormal condition of the Erectile Tissue.—Where, however, manifest impotence exists, which cannot be accounted for by the

12

the shape of small, indurated masses. The deposition of this lymph in the coverings of the penis causes them to lose their elasticity, the organ becomes non-erectile, and the man becomes incurably impotent.

Tubercular Affection of the Testes.—In addition to the other disorders we have already spoken of, impotence may arise, in delicate constitutions, from tubercles deposited in the testis itself or in the epididymis. Impotence is occasionally found arising from syphilitic deposits in the testes. It is partial or entire, according as one or both organs are more or less deeply implicated, and in proportion as the deposits have existed for a longer or shorter time. Orchitis may more or less interfere with the functions of the testes, but the impotence arising from the inflammation set up in the parenchymatous structure may rapidly subside, and the organ recover its full function. When, however, hard nodules remain in the epididymis, and in spite of treatment are persistent in both testicles, a grave suspicion may arise whether the patient will ever regain his virile powers; if, however, only one organ is affected, complete recovery may, as a rule, be expected. Each case must be judged by itself, and the prognosis will depend upon a variety of circumstances that cannot be noted in these pages.

PROGNOSIS.—When we remember the variety of complex and consentaneous actions which perfect sexual congress requires, it seems really astonishing that impotence should not be more common than it is.

To make coition complete, there must be—1. Excitement of the glans penis. 2. Suffusion of blood through the organ. 3. Contraction of the bulbo-cavernosi and ischio-cavernosi muscles. 4. Welling back of the blood of the bulb in the corpus spongiosum urethræ. 5. Compression of the dorsal vein of the penis by the anterior portion of the bulbo-cavernosi muscles. Now, if any one of these phenomena is checked or prevented, practical impotence is the necessary result. Thus, if the venous plexuses which make up the spongy portion of the urethra present varicose tumors, or if the muscle is enfeebled or paralyzed, the blood not arriving in sufficient quantity at the glans, the primitive ex-

portance in relation to his species. In consequence, the loss of virile power produces an effect more overpowering than that of honors, fortune, friends, or relatives; even the loss of liberty is as nothing compared to this internal and continual torture. Those who suffer from injustice or misfortune can accuse their enemies, society, chance, &c., and invent or retain the consciousness of not having deserved their lot; they have, moreover, the consolation of being able to complain, and the certainty of sympathy. But the impotent man[1] asserts that he can make a confidant of no one, that he can expect sympathy from no one. His misery is of a sort which cannot even inspire pity, and his greatest anxiety is lest any should penetrate his dismal secret." (Vol. iii, p. 119.)

DIAGNOSIS.—Before marriage, it has been supposed that it is very difficult for a medical man to decide whether an individual is truly impotent or not. Lallemand greatly exaggerates and indeed misrepresents the case, when he says that the power of easily maintaining perfect continence and entire quiescence of the sexual organs and desires "are fair grounds for presuming that there is little, if any, energy in the generative system, for if the semen was retained in the vesiculæ seminales it would produce from time to time energetic, or at least perceptible effects." (Vol. ii, p. 245.)

So vague a test as this can be hardly ever applied with safety. For instance, if a healthy man has his organs well developed, suffers only occasionally from emissions, has never abused his sexual powers, and is subject occasionally, in the early morning, to erections, then I should have no hesitation in saying that, although he may have been always continent, and may have found it easy to be so, there is, nevertheless, little doubt of his capability of performing the sexual act.

There are, however, other cases which do not admit of such ready solution, as the following instance shows. A middle-aged

---

[1] The belief, or rather assertion, of the patient, that he can make a confidant of no one is most untrue, as my profession are admitted to be ever ready to hold out their sympathy to the afflicted; and there are, I believe, few clergymen who would not sympathize fully with their distresses if the sufferers would but make a confidant of them.

probable than that a nervous man, who for the first time, meets a loose woman, goes to a strange house, and is frightened by the disgrace which may attend any exposure of his folly, should find himself unable to perform the act. The only greater misfortune that can befall him is to be deluded subsequently and consequently into consulting the advertising quacks. If he does not end his days in a lunatic asylum, he will be singularly fortunate.[1]

If however, real impotence is thought to exist, we must push our diagnosis further, and inquire whether it extends to the entire act of copulation, or only to some part of it, that is, whether the weakness depends upon something amiss in the acts of ERECTION, or EMISSION, or in the condition of the EJACULATED SEMEN, subjects which will be fully treated of in subsequent pages, as it is most important that the surgeon, in investigating the local symptoms, should discover which of these functions is imperfectly performed, otherwise he stands but a poor chance of relieving his patient's special complaint.

me, that in his youth he consulted an eminent London physician, who, though the ailment had no relation whatever to the sexual system, volunteered to say that it was bad for him to remain chaste : and in reply to some exclamation of surprise, explained that he must 'judge for himself how to act: the question of morality did not belong to the physician ; but, that *a man must not expect to be in health, if he neglected to exercise a natural function.*' " Mr. Newman goes on to say—" Different in basis, but equally formidable to morals, is the notion, that it is useless to struggle for the entire purity of young men ; and that their temporary unchastity (of course at the expense of women) is to be counted on. On all sides, a *despair of moral influences* is deplorably prevalent. It must be disowned, and a strict moral practice demanded : else, more and more, we shall see fatal acquiescence in a most destructive vice. The European Continent gives us most awful warning. On the whole, I find it impossible to resist the conviction, that in all ranks of the medical faculty there is at least a fraction (highly dangerous, if only a fraction), which actively preaches deadly immorality."—*The Relation of Physiology to Sexual Morals*, p. 23.

[1] As these pages were passing through the press a very lamentable case came under my notice. An officer returned from India, and attracted by the advertisement of a notorious quack, consulted him. After a great number of visits, intercourse with a woman of the town was recommended, and the first attempt was followed by chancre, and this by secondary symptoms. Before his victim escaped, the quack had obtained from him 1500*l.* Fortunately for himself, the patient sought other advice in time, and is now, I am happy to say, in a condition to perform his military duties efficiently.

lieved, and subsequently a stimulant given, we could understand the formula. Such should be the true method of effecting a cure; and I shall attempt, in the following pages, to indicate the principles which should guide its application. Had these principles been more generally followed, many of the invalids we meet with would have been rescued from much physical and mental suffering.

Cantharides have been employed against impotence. They form the basis of the *pastilles de Serail*, as well as of the numerous pills, pastes, and opiates which constitute in the East the principal commerce of all those who sell drugs. The Spanish fly enters largely into the *diavolini* and other aphrodisiac preparations still too much employed in India.

Lallemand protests strongly against the use of this dangerous stimulant.

"The effect," he says, "produced by cantharides on a healthy man, has induced persons to believe that they could restore virility lost from excesses. Thus, charlatans, and even many legitimate practitioners, have at all times prescribed cantharides as a traditional resource. For my own part, I have seldom met with an impotent person who has not had cause to regret using this drug. The greater proportion have not even experienced the momentary benefit which they had expected; and in many cases the erectile tissues have become smaller than in the habitual state of repose. Some few have experienced erections more or less energetic, which have lasted a longer or shorter period; but the loss of semen has exasperated the symptoms instantaneously, or very shortly afterwards."—Lallemand, vol. iii, p. 333.

No doubt can exist that the habitual employment of cantharides is prejudicial; but in the present day, when this substance is no longer given so indiscriminately as it was formerly, the surgeon may occasionally prescribe it with advantage. Thus, where the erection is feeble, when the fears of the patient exert much influence over his mind, or when there is doubt of his power to perform the copulative act, a few doses are very advisable. But after success, the remedy must be left off, for we do not want to excite the organs frequently, experience teaching us that the re-

If, however, I admit the value of this remedy in such cases, I must raise my voice against the indiscriminate and general employment of belts and other apparatus, so largely advertised. Hardly does a day pass but I find cases coming under my notice of patients wearing these appliances, who say they have derived no benefit, although they have worn them for months. Such a result is not surprising. If these batteries are efficient, they are always acting, and consequently are continually stimulating the sexual nerves. This, as I have above mentioned, has a most injurious effect.

It is one thing to rouse a lethargic constitution at periods when the stimulus is required, but quite another to keep the sexual organs in a constant state of nervous excitability. The consequence naturally follows that, at different and at long intervals, when the excitement is required, this valuable remedy ceases to exert any influence, and the most heart-rending effects are produced on the mind of the patient, who believing that a cure is impossible, relapses into a condition of desperation that no one can conceive, except those who have witnessed it. It is, moreover, difficult to rouse the nervous system a second time. The further objection to these batteries is that, as the patient can apply them himself, he does so at most inopportune moments, dispensing with the medical superintendence of the remedy which is necessary to secure a good result. I raise my voice most energetically against the public using either electricity or cantharides, without first taking the opinion of a medical man, as to whether such stimulants are applicable to the case, and also as to the dose, and the frequency and time of application.

Marriage has been classed among the remedies for the slighter affections of the sexual organs; and if I may credit the statements of patients, medical men, on being consulted, in the most off-hand manner, without inquiring into the particular symptoms or probable cause of the supposed impotency, at once say, " Oh! you are only nervous; go and get married—a wife will cure you!"

In the milder cases, and in the instances where the patient only slightly suffers from too frequent nocturnal emissions, but in other respects is in good health, no advice can be better, and I am only too glad to corroborate it.

Amidst all the important questions, however, that come before a medical man, I know of none which require more tact and knowledge than this :—" Am I in a condition to marry?" On the one hand you have, perhaps, the very timid, nervous individual, previously depicted in these pages, who may or may not have exaggerated his weaknesses until neither he nor his medical adviser can exactly say what is his condition. Often even in the slighter cases it requires all the knowledge acquired by long practice to arrive at a just conclusion as to what is real, what fanciful in a patient's narrative. It is, in short, most difficult to say, off-hand, in such cases, whether a man may or may not marry. I must admit I am always disposed to take the sanguine view of the probabilities, as experience teaches me that the majority of adults are liable to perform the sexual act. It is a calamitous thing for a healthy adult to be told by a scientific man, unless on clear and sufficient ground, that he is so far impotent that he should not marry.[1]

Although a professional man may almost invariably give this favorable opinion, he should recollect that the very fact of its being thought worth while to consult him affords *primâ facie* evidence that *the patient* feels that something is amiss ; and experience teaches me that the healthy adult does not ask the opinion of a medical man without having pretty good reason to suspect that he is wanting in virile power. So convinced am I of this, that when a patient consults me on the advisability of

[1] It not unfrequently happens that a young man, in consulting his doctor, appeals to his feelings, and says, "Tell me the worst; I am ready to hear the statement that I may not marry, but do not let me marry and repent of it, and make two people wretched—at present I have only myself to care for, and I could bear the worst opinion you can give of me." I may say that after thirty years' experience, I have hardly ever found myself compelled to pronounce a young man, otherwise healthy, to be impotent who held such language as this. I can most conscientiously state that in nine cases out of ten such complainants are only diffident men, who belong to the susceptible class so often depicted in these pages. I may lay it down as a general rule that those who are anxious to marry may do so without any dread of being impotent.

marriage I enter fully into details, and inquire into his antecedents. I generally find that he is not only suffering from too frequent emissions, but also that his fears depend upon facts which he is not all at once ready to disclose. The result of these inquiries too often proves that the patient, although a continent man, goaded by his fears, has made one or two unsuccessful attempts at sexual intercourse.

The pleasure with which these patients receive the announcement that they may marry must be seen to be appreciated, yet they can hardly believe that the opinion is unbiassed. As I have said elsewhere, diffidence is a marked characteristic of these men, and they again and again ask, "Are you not taking too favorable view of my case?" They display the most unselfish feelings, and reassert that they could bear their own miserable state of existence, but entreat the surgeon not to sacrifice the woman. As I have said above, most of these are not cases of true impotence, and it would be indeed be a grievous error on the part of a medical man to condemn such patients to a state of celibacy, and if the appropriate treatment described at page 77 be followed, in a very short time a marked recovery may be observed, which surely progresses, until at length the patient becomes satisfied of his healthy condition. I am in the habit of assuring such patients that no one more than myself is convinced of the danger of recommending a man to marry who is physically unfit to do so. I fully agree in the truth of what the professor of Montpelier has nobly observed, "What has the young girl, who is thus sacrificed to an egotistical calculation, done, that she should be condemned to the existence that awaits her? Who has the right to regard her as a therapeutic agent, and to risk thus lightly her future prospects, her repose, and the happiness of the remainder of her life?"

"Until a man has contracted these indissoluble bonds, impotence the most complete can compromise the future of no one.

"It is precisely because marriage is the most sacred bond for individuals, as well as the most important for society, and because an iron law renders it indissoluble, that it is rational as well as moral not to contract it without the certainty that it will be perfect and complete." (Vol. iii, p. 470.)

I can, however, affirm that in practice I have never known an instance of this sort of martyrdom where my sanction to a marriage has been previously asked and granted.

It often happens that when a medical man thinks it desirable for a patient to marry, his advice is frustrated by other considerations. In many cases, the patient is too young ; in other instances, where sexual abuse has been indulged in, or nocturnal emission has been frequent, the dislike to marriage is such that every woman is alike distasteful to the sufferer, and we must first improve the patient's state of health.

Those nervous, hypochondriacal people who, from a bad conscience, a weak frame, the effects of depressed health, or some wild ideas of the possible requirements of the young lady,[1] on the subject of which all well-brought up English maidens are ignorant, fancy that they are unfit to undertake the rational duties, of husbands and fathers, should be encouraged to marry and be happy.

In conclusion, I must add my firm conviction that when the surgeon has improved the health of these self-accusing nervous men, nothing is so likely to establish a permanent cure and therefore conduce to the happiness of individuals as marriage. But it will be well for the medical man, who thus advises marriage, to impress on the patient how necessary it will be that he indulge in no form of excess.   Organs that have been temporarily weakened require to be exercised with great moderation.

SECOND DIVISION.

THE SEXUAL ACT, ITS PHYSIOLOGY AND DISORDERS.

WE come now to the second of the main divisions of this part of the work.   And first of all I propose to consider the several conditions and acts which go to make up the entire act of coition. 1st, I shall describe them as they occur in health or normally ;

[1] See page 162 in corroboration of this statement.

and 2dly, I shall point out in what way they may occur abnormally, preventing or interfering with the complete performance of the copulative act.

To the physiologist, but more especially to the medical man engaged in practice, a knowledge of the more intimate causes of potence or impotence is most important, and hardly less so to the thousands who suffer in one way or another, from some of the many causes that may hamper, or entirely prevent, the exercise of the reproductive functions.

To the due performance of copulation three things are indispensable—namely, 1st, *erection of the penis;* 2d, *the power of emission or ejaculation;* and 3d, *a due amount of well-formed semen;* all which it will be necessary to treat of in the three following chapters.

CHAPT. I.—ERECTION.

In pursuance of the plan which we have hitherto followed, we shall divide this chapter into two parts, in the first describing the normal act and its essential conditions, and in the second the disorders to which erection may be subject.

PART I.

NORMAL ERECTION, OR CONDITIONS ESSENTIAL TO IT.

This external sign of virility, as Buffon calls Erection, depends chiefly on the existence in the organ of certain tissues known as *erectile tissues.* Let us see what the most recent anatomical investigations have taught us regarding these important structures. The following remarks are extracted from the seventh edition of Kirkes' " Physiology," by M. Baker.

" ERECTILE TISSUES.—The instances of greatest variation in the quantity of blood contained at different times in the same organs are found in certain structures, which, under ordinary cir-

under the same muscles, and the veins of the bulb are subject to the compression of the bulbo-cavernosi. (See *Krause*, lxxx, 1837; *Köbelt*, cxxvii and xxv, 1843, p. 58.)

"Erection results from the distension of the venus plexuses with blood. The principal exciting cause in the erection of the penis is nervous irritation originating in the part itself,[1] or derived from the brain or spinal cord. The nervous influence is communicated to the penis by the pubic nerves, which ramify in its vascular tissue, and Günther (xcvi, 1828, p. 364) has observed that, after their division in the horse the penis is no longer capable of erection. It affords a good example of the subjection of the circulation in an individual organ, to the influence of the nerves, but the mode in which they excite a greater influx of blood is not with certainty known.

"The most probable explanation is that offered by Professor Kölliker,[2] who ascribes the distension of the venous plexuses to the influence of organic muscular fibres, which he finds in abundance in the corpora cavernosa of the penis, from the bulb to the glans, also in the clitoris and other parts capable of erection. While the erectile organs are flaccid and at rest, these contractile fibres exercise an amount of pressure on the plexuses of vessels distributed amongst them sufficient to prevent their distension with blood. But when, through the influence of their nerves, these parts are stimulated to erection, the action of these fibres is suspended, and the plexuses thus liberated from pressure yield

---

[1] "The glans penis," says Köbelt, "is the principal point of reunion of the sensitive nerves of the virile organ, no other part which it regulates can be compared with it in this respect. In respect to richness in nerves, the glans penis yields to no other part of the economy, not even the organs of sense." (Köbelt, loc. cit., p. 10.)

[2] Kölliker says, "Erection is caused, as I have shown ('Würzb. Verh.' Bd. ii), by a relaxation of the muscular elements in the *trabeculæ* of the cavernous and spongy bodies, and of the *tunica media* of the arteries of those parts, in consequence of which the tissue, like a sponge which has been compressed, expands, and becomes filled with blood. The rigidity ensues so soon as the muscles are completely relaxed and the sinuses filled to the utmost, without there being any necessity that the return of the blood should be impeded and the circulation stopped. It ceases when the muscles again contract, the venous spaces become narrowed, and the blood is expressed from them."

13

to the distended force of the blood, which, probably, at the same time, arrives in greater quantity, owing to a simultaneous dilatation of the parts ; and thus the plexuses become filled, and remain so until the stimulus to erection subsides, when the organic muscular fibres again contract, and so gradually expel the excess of blood from the previously distended vessels."—*Kirkes*, p. 142.

In speaking of the nerves, Müller says : " The corpora cavernosa of the penis and urethra are provided in greater part with nerves of organic life, whereas the glans penis, very sensitive as it is, receives nerves exclusively sensitive."—*Müller*, "*Ueber die Organischen Nerven der erectilen Männlichen Geschlechtsorgane,*" &c., p. 44.

" The arteries of erectile organs present a special disposition, which strikes one at once.   At first (as Müller has shown) the arterial trunks in the bulb and at the roots of the corpora cavernosa do not divide in the usual way into dichotomic branches, but are surrounded on all sides by bunches of vessels which arise, from three to ten in number, from a short common trunk.   These vessels are not mere short diverticula, but traverse for some distance the large sinuses of the central portion of the corpora cavernosa and of the bulb, and penetrate, after numerous subdivisions and anastomoses, especially about the periphery, the muscular trabeculæ.   After traversing these fibres, the arteries pass to the surface through slit-like openings ; but from their origin to their termination in the muscular fibres, the vessels from the arterial branches are twisted on themselves, in abrupt and closely compressed spiral folds, interlacing, entwining, and anastomosing, so as to form a sort of vascular tangle, and this, unlike any simple flexions which a slight distension suffices to obliterate, persists during even complete erection, and closely resembles a beautiful network."—*Rouget, Professeur agrégé à la Faculté de Médecine de Paris*, "*Journ. de Physiologie,*" tom. i, p. 881.

Köbelt describes erection as follows:—"Thus, on the one hand, the glans penis, endowed as it is with sensibility, and, on the other hand, the *irritable* muscular apparatus of the bulb, act and react upon one another as reciprocal exciting causes. The glans penis, when excited, reacts on the bulb, which sends more and more blood—the exciting material—towards it. Each new rush of blood to the glans exalts its sensibility ; the bulbo-cavernosus muscle, *irritated* in its turn, progressively accelerates its contractions, in order to satisfy the requirements of the glans, which also increases more and more, till at last, by alternate actions, the entire apparatus reaches its highest point of excitement. At this moment a new series of secondary reflex phenomena is suddenly produced between the glans penis and the muscles which produce evacuation of the vesiculæ seminales, these muscles become excited, a spermatic ejaculation is produced, and at this point the currents of exchange cease, the special function is accomplished, and the organ, as soon as nature has gained her end, returns to its ordinary state of repose and vegetative life."—*Köbelt*, loc. cit., p. 39.

Rouget has lately given us his views as to the way in which erection takes place. Contraction commences in front of the bulb and the root of the cavernous body, or at least at their margin. He supposes that " the distension of the vesiculæ seminales is the first cause of natural erection. The latter commences by a species of spasm, which, developing itself in the muscular apparatus of the generative system, is transmitted *de proche en proche* to the bundles of the root of the cavernous body and the bulb, and tends to propagate itself to the whole extent of the penis. The obstacle to the course of blood in the veins of the plexus of *Santorini*, imposed by the first muscular contractions, has for its immediate effect the dilatation of the areola of the cavernous bodies by the blood ; and the tension of the liquid struggles energetically against the muscular tonicity up to the moment when, ejaculation being accomplished, spasm ceases little by little in the same situations where it began ; the circulation then becoming free, muscular contraction gets the better of the tension of the blood, and partially drives on this liquid. The organ itself then gradually resumes its natural dimensions."

These recent researches, then, seem to demonstrate that the muscular contractions, the effect of which is to hamper the

when the penis is introduced into the vagina of the bitch, its body becomes suddenly enlarged, and the animal is thus unable to withdraw from connection for a long time. This, according to Richerand, depends upon the absence of visiculæ seminales in the dog; and as the semen passes only drop by drop, impregnation would not occur had not nature ordained such prolonged copulation. This appears very probable.

In some animals, as in the monkeys, the bats, the carnivora, the rodentia, and the balænidæ among cetaceans, erection is further assisted by a bone which is imbedded in the substance of the male organ, of which it forms a considerable part. Where this bone exists the corpora cavernosa are proportionably small, and the fibrous walls of the penis are confounded with its periosteal covering.

That the erect penis should fill the vagina and distend it seems necessary to the full excitement of the female sexual feelings. It appears from the following account given by Rymer Jones, in his "General Outline of the Animal Kingdom," that nature has given to certain classes of animals an apparatus which deserves the attention of the surgeon; he says—

"In the guinea-pig no one will be disposed to deny that the penis is an instrument of excitement. It is strengthened by a flat bone that reaches forward as far as the extremity of the glans, beneath which is the termination of the urethra; but behind and below the orifice of this canal is the opening of the pouch, wherein are lodged two long, horny spikes. When the member is erect the pouch alluded to becomes everted, and the spikes are protruded externally to a considerable length. Both the everted pouch and the entire surface of the glans are, moreover, covered densely with sharp spines or hooklets; and as though even all this were not sufficient to produce the needful irritation, still further back there are, in some species, two short and strong horny saws appended to the sides of the organ. From this terrible armature of the male cavys it would be only natural to expect some corresponding peculiarity in the female parts; but, however inexplicable it may appear, the female vagina offers no uncommon structure." (p. 835.)

PART II.

ABNORMAL ERECTION AND DISORDERS AFFECTING ERECTION.

HAVING described normal erection and its essential conditions, it remains for us to consider a few of the more frequent perversions or morbid states affecting this function, and for the convenience of description I have treated of them under the separate sections of—

    I. SLOW ERECTION.
    II. ERECTION NOT LASTING LONG ENOUGH.
    III. IMPERFECT ERECTION.
    IV. IRREGULAR ERECTION.
    V. NON-ERECTION.
    VI. PRIAPISM, OR PERMANENT ERECTION.
    VII. SATYRIASIS.

SECT. I.—SLOW ERECTION.

This peculiarity occurs in animals as well as men. I observed it in horses when, in 1862, I had the opportunity of visiting the well-organised horse-breeding establishment of Mr. Blenkiron in company with Professor Spooner. A chestnut stallion in particular, aged and somewhat fat, was remarkable in this respect. He required to be walked about and around the mare before any erection took place, and in mounting the act lasted rather longer than is usual with other stallions.

This sluggishness, which is often rather a congenital peculiarity than a disorder, sometimes causes alarm when it exists in man. I have often been consulted by persons telling me that erection is very tardy, and requesting some stimulus for the purpose of expediting the act. Of course the invariable reply to such a request is that it would be very dangerous to interfere. The best means of allaying the anxiety of such patients is to explain to them the real cause of the symptom. If it arises from temperament, there is nothing to be alarmed at. Lethargic heavy men experience this symptom just as the too susceptible suffer from the contrary one of too rapid erection and emission. A little seasonable advice and sympathy may often in such cases prevent much unhappiness and misunderstanding. Fitting medical treatment, moreover, can often insure some amendment, although of course nothing can alter the character and temperament of the man.

SECT. II.—ERECTION NOT LASTING LONG ENOUGH.

This is one of the disordered varieties of erection which is not unfrequent, and it gives rise to a great deal of annoyance. A man finds himself potent; he wakes with erections of a morning, and finds that they occur also under excitement, but to his chagrin discovers that when he attempts sexual intercourse the erection fails, and the act is imperfectly performed, because the organ all at once suddenly collapses.

In the opinion of the patient this is a very serious matter, but fortunately the medical man is able to give a very reassuring opinion. On investigating the causes of such failures, it will be found that this state of things depends upon causes that can be in most cases easily removed. I have known this form of disorder arise in many instances from the patient waiting too long. Erection will last but a certain time, this of course varying in different persons, and in some it can be maintained only a short time. Persons so circumstanced should not dally, otherwise failure is likely to occur. The treatment in these cases is of the simplest kind; I advise the patient not to attempt to repeat the act for twelve or twenty-four hours, or until strong desire recurs; then let him take care not to delay the act, and he will find that the erection will suffice. The occurrence, however, particularly if it occur in married men, should prove to them that age is advancing, and that the sexual power thus gives evidence of failure. To the prudent man, under these circumstances, it is a sign that he must economize his resources, and not give way to his passions, particularly if in youth he has committed excesses.

tion was not attended with much benefit. In this instance W— had a slight curvature in the back, and he mentioned that in early life he had suffered from disease of the spine, with loss of motion in the lower extremities; from this he recovered by exten- tion. He likewise confessed that he had been a great masturba- tor. I did not, however, ascertain if the affection of the spine preceded or followed the indulgence of this habit.

Writers on anatomy and physiology have given very little in- formation which will assist the surgeon in the treatment of these cases; however, Köbelt thinks that indolent erections (that is to say, those which we notice in drunken people, in children, in old men and persons of debilitated constitutions) never extend be- yond the corpora cavernosa of the penis, and they never affect the passive organ, that is to say, the glans penis and corpus spongiosum urethræ. The glans particularly, in such cases, never attains its full size, except when the other subordinate parts have been previously in a state of complete turgescence; it will be hence understood why in certain conditions (notwithstand- ing the complete rigidity of the body of the penis), neither orgasm nor seminal ejaculation can be produced.—*Köbelt*, loc. cit., p. 60.

In many of these cases, where the imperfect erection has, in my opinion, depended upon want of support to the vessels, I have found great benefit from binding up the penis with strips of plaster, on the same principle that we treat varicose veins in the lower extremities, and I have been singularly successful. The occasional passing of a bougie, and even cauterization, has been likewise attended with remarkably successful results. In other instances galvanism, and even local stimulants, with the precaution mentioned at page 187, have proved very successful in my hands.

SECT. IV.—IRREGULAR ERECTION.

Again, the erection may be abnormal in nature and most pain- fully distort the penis while it lasts.

In March, 18—, a middle-aged gentleman called on me, and

My reply to such a man is, "be thankful that your studies are not interfered with by sensual thoughts." I advise him to continue to work hard, but not to omit regular and daily gymnastic exercise. Observation teaches me that, after this long rest of the organs, the seminal fluid will be formed in great abundance as soon as the brain shall have ceased its inordinate demands upon the blood.

The antagonism of the nervous and generative system has not escaped the notice of writers on population. Spencer says—"Thus, the fact that intense mental application, involving great waste of the nervous tissues, and a corresponding consumption of nervous matter for their repair, is accompanied by a cessation in the production of sperm-cells, gives strong support to the hypothesis that the sperm-cells consists essentially of neurine. And this becomes yet clearer on finding that the converse fact is true, that undue production of sperm-cells involves cerebral inactivity. Throughout the vertebrate tribes the degree of fertility varies inversely as the development of the nervous system."

SECT. VI.—PRIAPISM, OR PERMANENT ERECTION.

Erection again, instead of being absent or imperfect, may be only too frequently and readily excited and too persistent. This is what is called *priapism*. Fortunately for human nature, this terrible and humiliating condition, in its full extent, is by no means common. Every now and then, nevertheless, we meet with cases where, instead of the erection only lasting a few minutes,—the male organ again resuming its usual relaxed condition,—the penis will, if the statements of patients can be believed, remain erect either permanently or during long periods.

It is to the condition of the spinal cord and brain that we must look for the source of this phenomenon. These, after all, are the primary sources of sexual excitement, and on them depend the entire processes of erection and ejaculation. Lallemand relates a case in which a patient could produce ejaculation by striking his head with his knuckles. Depuytren has long since

pline or self-constraint—which there was little need to inculcate,—but simply physical cleanliness, to accustom the part to feel water. I told him that, if ablution produced sexual feelings at first, not to mind, but to persevere, as these would cease immediately the morbid irritability had been got rid of. As soon as the external sensitiveness had been overcome, I gradually passed an instrument, and discovered the greatest morbid irritability of the urethra I ever met with. This, however, gradually declined, and the tendency to priapism disappeared.

The medical man, however, must not expect always to produce so speedy a cure as this. Indeed, as regards the treatment of this troublesome ailment, I must admit I have been much disappointed with most remedies, though I have tried nearly all those that have from time to time been recommended. Some years ago Sir Charles Locock made known, at a meeting of the Royal Medical and Chirurgical Society, what he considered a very important fact with regard to the treatment of some forms of epilepsy. He stated that in cases of hysterical epilepsy in young women connected with sexual excitement, and recurring at the periods of menstruation, he had found the bromide of potassium, in doses of from five to ten grains, remarkably efficacious. Of fifteen cases in which he had tried it, it had failed in only one. Sir Charles attributed the good effects of the bromide to its power of diminishing sexual excitement. In consequence of this recommendation I experimented with this salt pretty largely and in very various doses. In some instances, I thought I noticed beneficial effects, but in other cases no amendment followed; and I now depend upon local remedies and those applications which more especially influence the spinal cord, irritation of which seems particularly to promote priapism.

SECT. VII.—SATYRIASIS.

Erection again may not only be morbidly frequent and persistent, but connected with a maniacal sensuality that is one of the most awful visitations to which humanity can be subject.

tation of the cerebellum exists to a degree quite sufficient to account for the most painful and deplorable symptoms.

Mr. Dunn, in 1849, brought before the Medical and Chirurgical Society an interesting case of death from apoplexy, attended with a softened pulpy state of the right hemisphere of the cerebellum, in the midst of which was an apoplectic clot of the size of a pullet's egg. The patient's wife had observed that he had been subject to a constant desire for sexual intercourse. In the discussion which followed, Dr. Carpenter referred to a case mentioned to him some years ago by Mr. Turley, of Worcester, in which a man advanced in life became the subject of satyriasis to such a degree, that he would even practice masturbation in the presence of females, and after death a tumour of the size of a split pea was found on the pons varolii. (See "Lancet," vol. i, 1849, p. 329.)

A physician in the west of London was recently called in to attend a powerful man, of between fifty and sixty, who exhibited every indication of approaching homicidal mania. He found, on inquiry, that the present fit had been preceded by an extravagant indulgence in connection with his wife. The proper remedies were used, the patient became somewhat calmed, and the wife was solemnly warned on no account to permit any renewal of intercourse. She was a weak woman, and from time to time yielded, each indulgence being followed by a fresh outbreak on the part of the patient. At last, after a series of excesses, the homicidal fury broke out in full force, when, with considerable danger, the party was secured and conveyed to a lunatic asylum.

SMALL SIZE OF PENIS.

Before quitting the subject of erection, I must remark *on the size of the intromittent organ.* In the negro it is proverbially large, but, as in the case of whites also, who have the same pecu-

CHAPT. II.—EMISSIONS.

Emission is the second of the requisites specified at page 191 to complete intercourse.

PART I.

NORMAL FUNCTIONS, OR CONDITIONS AFFECTING EMISSION.

It is thus described by Kirkes:—" The emission of semen is a reflex act, and as such is governed by the spinal cord. The irritation of the glans penis conducted to the spinal cord, and thence reflected excites the successive and co-ordinate contracting of the muscular fibres of the vasa deferentia and vesiculæ seminales, of the accelerator urinæ and other muscles of the urethra; and a forcible expulsion of semen takes place over which the mind has little or no control, and which in cases of paraplegia may be unfelt."—*7th Edition*, p. 506.

Valentin adds:—" This effect may be artificially produced in recently killed animals. The semen reaches the inferior and glandular part of the vas deferens. It then traverses the urethra to the orifice of the glans, when it is ejaculated with a force which in vigorous men can expel it to a distance of many feet."—*Valentin translated by Brinton*, p. 625.

The semen, however, as emitted, is not the semen as it is secreted in the testes. It may be said, while in the testes, to be in little more than a rudimentary state. When ejaculated it is a highly elaborated secretion. None, in fact, amongst the various secretions of the body seems to require so much time to mature. Not only have cells to be formed and thrown off, as in the case of other secretions, but, after they are liberated in the tubercles of the testis, nuclei have to divide, nucleoli to multiply, and each division of the nucleoli to become, through a gradual adolescence, an adult spermatozoon. When thus prepared it is passed down the spermatic cords to the vesiculæ seminales. The vesiculæ,

14

a great proportion of involuntary muscular fibre, and there is also a large admixture of involuntary fibre in the proper parietes of the tube. In the elephant the vesiculæ seminales present, on the outer and anterior aspect, a peculiar muscle rising from the neck and middle part of the sac, and spreading out over the upper part, which can contract the cavity and expel the contents.

In animals that have a rutting season the vesiculæ seminales, as well as the testicles, prostate gland, &c., are exceedingly small during the period of rest, and enlarge enormously and rapidly previously to the season of rut.

The semen, before it is ejaculated, is not only matured, as has been described, but is mixed with the secretion of the vesiculæ seminales and with that of the prostate. The object of this dilution seems to be to render it more fluid, and thus more capable of passing easily along its course. As soon as the thick mucus of the vesiculæ seminales is squeezed out and meets the semen, the mixture becomes much more fluid than either of its component parts. Indeed, if the mucus is exposed to the air before the semen is added, it becomes almost solid.

It is owing to the abundance of these other secretions that ejaculation takes place after the removal of the testicles. A striking instance of this came under my notice a few years ago. On the 4th of January, 1859, Mr. Holthouse removed both testes from a man in consequence of his suffering from epilepsy. The case created a good deal of discussion at the time; and as the patient entered another hospital for a different complaint, a medical friend, thinking I should like to know the result, sent him to me, and on the 26th of March, 1859,—that is, nearly three months after the castration,—I ascertained the following particulars :

Within the week following the removal of the testes this man had two emissions. Since then three more emissions occurred, the last on the 2d of March; that is, two months after the operation. At the time I saw him he appeared in no way distressed in mind, and I could note no symptoms betokening him a monomaniac. He complained of a frequent desire to make water. I tested the urine, but found it natural.

Sir Astley Cooper, in his observations on "Diseases of the Testes," p. 54, mentions having removed both testes from a man. Four days afterwards the patient had an emission, which appeared upon his linen."

"For nearly the first twelve months he stated that he had emissions *in coitu*, or that he had the sensations of emission. That then he had erections and coitus at distant intervals, but without the sensation of emission. After two years he had erections very rarely and very imperfectly, and they generally ceased immediately upon the attempt at coitus. Ten years after the operation he said he had during the past year been only once connected.

"Twenty-eight years after the operation, he stated that for years he had seldom any erection, and then that it was imperfect; that he had no emissions from the first year of the operation; that he had for many years only a few times attempted coitus, but unsuccessfully; that he had once or twice dreams of desire, and a sensation of emission, but without the slightest appearance of it. The penis was shrivelled and wasted. He was in the habit of shaving once a week, and sometimes twice. His voice, naturally rather feeble, remained as at the time of the operation."

Of the persistence of sexual desires, and to a certain extent sexual power, we read in Juvenal:

> "Sunt quas eunuchi imbelles ac mollia semper
> Oscula delectent ac desperatio barbæ
> Et quod abortivo non est opus."

Köbelt imagines that excision of the glans penis would destroy all desire, as it is the rendezvous of the sensitive nerves which excite venereal desires.

That this statement is not borne out by facts, is clearly proved by the case in my own practice, related at page 135, where the glans penis had been destroyed, and yet the patient fully performed all his marital duties. We have also the experience of practical shepherds, who find that the removal of the "worms," as they call the point of the penis in the ram, does not prevent the ram from attempting connection. Division of the public nerves, however, seems infallibly to annihilate all sexual feeling, and to destroy at once the power and the desire of connection. Günther observes :

"After division of the nerves of the penis (nervi dorsalis penis) the most powerful and erotic stallion appears almost at once to be more completely deprived of every sexual feeling than he could possibly be after castration."—*Günther* "*Untersuchungen und Erfahrungen im Gebiete der Anatomie, Physiologie, und Thierarzenei-Kunde,*" *Hanover*, 1837, § 153.

EFFECT OF EMISSION IN THE MALE.—Emission in healthy males is attended with spasmodic excitement, followed by temporary nervous prostration. Lallemand calls this excitement *ébranlement nerveux epileptiforme.* This is seen in a very exaggerated form in the buck rabbit, who, after every copulation, may be noticed to fall on his side in a sort of epileptic fit; the whites of his eyes are turned up; he gives several spasmodic twitches with his hind legs, and lies panting for some moments, until the nervous system recovers itself.

There are some men in whom this sort of epileptiform orgasm takes place every time connection is indulged in. Napoleon I. is said to have been subject to epilepsy when, resting from his great labors, he indulged in sexual intercourse. No doubt can exist that deaths which have occurred in houses of ill-fame, as well as on the marriage couch, have arisen from this cause acting upon highly susceptible organizations. Entomological works abound with cases in which the male dies after the act of copulation. The following, which reads almost like romance, may be explained, perhaps, by this epileptiform attack killing the frail insect. It is a brief history of the establishment and growth of a colony of termite ants, as related by Burmeister.

"At the termination of the hot season, the young males and females quit the nest, and appear upon the surface of the earth, where they swarm in innumerable hosts, and pair. The busied workers then convey a chosen male and female back into the dwelling, and imprison them in the central royal cell, the entrances to which they decrease, and guard. Through these apertures the imprisoned pair then receive the nutriment they require.

notions on these matters. They believed that emission was the actual passage of brain down the spinal cord ; and we find them speaking of connection being followed by the *stillicidium cerebri*.

Hippocrates says : "The humors enter into a sort of fermentation, which separates what is most precious and most balsamic, and this part thus separated from the rest is carried by the spinal marrow to the generative organs."—DE GENITURA, *Foesieus*, p. 231.

This popular notion is not yet extinct. It is not long since I heard one man of the world coolly asserting to another, his entire belief that Lord——, a noted old libertine, was killing himself by inches ; that he had long sinced ceased to emit semen, and under unnatural excitement the substance of the brain was now passing away in the venereal orgasm, as was proved by the great nervous depression which was known to follow each sexual effort. The narrator moreover asserted most confidently that his lordship was aware of the fact ;·but, in spite of all remonstrance, no sooner did the old debauchee recover from the effects of one loss, than he incurred another.

Tabes dorsalis (apparently the ancient term for what the moderns call spermatorrhœa) is described by old writers as wasting of the spinal cord. So late as the time of Richerand, we find him, in his " Physiology," seriously asking his readers "if the nervous depression which follows connection depends upon the fatigue of the organs, or, as some metaphysicians have believed, is it caused by the confused and indistinct notion that the soul takes of its own destruction ?"

M. Parise also, in his valuable book on the diseases of old age, uses figurative but no less erroneous expressions to the same effect, which he has gleaned from the old writers.

"Semen is life itself under a fluid form—the vital principle condensed and perceptible. Camus said it was composed of microscopical brains directly emanating from the great brain. The ancients considered this liquid as a discharge from the spinal marrow and brain, and called it cerebri stillicidium."

"Its importance is demonstrated by the fact that the smallest quantity contains life in activity, and can communicate it ; that its presence and its secretion impress the organization with an extra quantity of force and energy, whereas repeated loss of it ennervates and rapidly wears out the body. Nothing costs the economy so much as the production of semen, and its forced ejaculation. It has been calculated that an ounce of semen was equivalent to forty ounces of blood. According to Bichat, the secretion of sperm is an inverse proportion to the secretion of fat; and we at once see the reason, semen is the essence of the whole individual. Hence Fernel has said, 'totus homo semen est.' It is the balm of life—one of its best and most powerful stimulants. That which gives life is intended for its preservation." (Reveillé-Parise, "De la Vieilesse," p. 415.)

Of course these alarming statements are not such as modern science can at all indorse. Nevertheless it should be remembered that the semen, as I have pointed out above, is a highly organized fluid, requiring the expenditure of much vital force in its elaboration and its expulsion. Even in the strongest adult, and much more in the youth or the weakly man, the whole of the functions connected with it are most vital and important—the last that should be abused.

PART II.

DISORDERS AFFECTING EMISSION.

WE have now to consider the disorders that may complicate or interfere with the ejaculatory part of the sexual act. It has been generally supposed that the loss of semen was the sole cause of sexual debility in the male. That such is not the case is proved by the nervous depression coming on in young children from sexual excitement before they can be said to secrete semen. Similar nervous exhausting effects are noticed in women, who do not secrete any such fluid, but merely mucus,[1] and yet may ex-

---

[1] No woman, any more than any other female animal, secretes or loses semen, or anything analogous to it during the sexual orgasm. The spent secretion contains no spermatozoa. What passes, if examined under the mi-

perience the nervous orgasm or spasm which acts as harmfully on them, when much indulged in, as on males.   The immediate cause of this nervous depression has, within the last few years, excited a good deal of attention ; and I, in common with many modern writers, have come to the conclusion that there is a good deal of evidence now existing which shows that shocks constantly received and frequently repeated on the great ganglionic centres may produce irritation in them, and thus cause many of the ob- scure forms of disease to which we have hitherto failed in discov- ering a key.   If there is any cause which is likely more than another to produce undue excitement of the ganglionic system, it is the too frequent repetition of acts involving this nervous orgasm.

It has been clearly proved by Brachet that if the solar plexus and semilunar ganglion in an animal be irritated, it will, as soon as the parts become inflamed, express feelings of suffering. When the communication is cut off between these ganglia and the spinal cord, all symptoms of pain or irritation of the ganglia cease.

Hence we should infer, I think, that undue excitement of the generative functions may set up irritation of these ganglia, and

croscope, consists of mucus or the debris of epithelium.   Nevertheless, as an effect of long-continued, and often repeated sexual shocks, women may ex- ceptionally—feeble as their sexual tendencies are compared with men's—be- come subject to epileptiform attacks, and various nervous affections, as well as local affections of the uterus, direct consequences of sexual excesses.   The womb, as has been well observed, is the centre round which women's sentient feelings radiate.   No one who has treated a large number of women laboring under uterine affections, but must have been struck with the haggard feverish pinched cast of countenance which too often characteristically denotes the existence of long-standing uterine affections.   In every way it resembles the look of the young libertine who has given way to a long-continued course of sexual excesses ; and the long lank hair of the enfeebled delicate girl-like boy tends often to make the delusion more perfect.   I had the painful duty lately of inspecting some photographs of boys who had for some time minis- tered to the depravity of the vilest men, and the lens had but too truly de- picted, and perhaps exaggerated, the hang-dog look which these youthful miscreants exhibited ; but I must admit that there were other portraits of youths who presented all the external symptoms of perfect blooming health, and could not be distinguished from ordinary well-conditioned young men.

portions. And it seems not improbable that these states are to be ascribed to the impairments of texture, which are naturally produced in the exercise of muscles, being in these instances unrepaired. It is certain that in the natural exercise of a muscle its composition and texture are, in however small a measure, changed; many of the results of the change have been traced by chemical analysis; fatigue is the sensation we have of the changed state of the muscles or its nerves; and the state is one of impairment, for the muscle has lost power. In health, and the natural course of events, the repair of the thus impaired muscle is accomplished during the repose which follows exercise. But, if due repose be not allowed, the impairments may accumulate, and the muscles may become gradually weaker, so as to need greater stimulus for the fulfilment of their ordinary work; and at length, in some instances, they may even lose the power of repairing themselves during repose. In these instances they are the subjects of the ‘progressive muscular atrophy.’

"Now, although the very nature and products of the changes that ensue in nervous organs during their exercise are less well known than are those that ensue in muscles, yet the occurrence of such changes is certain; some of them are traced by analysis; they are similarly felt by fatigue; similarly repaired in repose. And it seems a fair analogy which suggests that the loss of nervous power, and especially the paraplegia, that may follow long-continued sexual excess, are due to changes parallel with those that are witnessed in the progressive muscular atrophy after excessive muscular exercises—the softening and wasting of the paraplegic cord being a process of fatty and wasting degeneration essentially similar to that traced in muscles.

"In the progressive muscular atrophy, the wasting or other degeneration of the muscles generally proceeds, in course of time, to muscles more and more distant from those first affected after over-work; by similar process, the degeneration of the spinal cord may extend far from the part first affected in consequence of its over-exercise in the sexual acts.

"It is taken for granted here that the act of copulation and emission is associated with what may be regarded as violent exercise of the spinal cord; and this cannot reasonably be doubted. But I have also no doubt that cases of paraplegia may be sometimes seen in which the excessive exercise of the cord has been in its participation in violent and long-continued voluntary muscular actions, especially in excessive walking, running, and other such acts.

"In what is said above, I have had in view only the cases of *gradual* loss of nervous power due to excessive sexual acts. Where the loss is *rapid*, it may be due to inflammation (associated as that process is with rapid degeneration) of the nervous organs. But here, also, the parallel with muscles will hold; for an excessively exercised muscle not unfrequently becomes inflamed, and its inflammation may very quickly lead to its wasting or other degeneration, and its corresponding loss of power.

"I cannot guess why excessive sexual acts should be followed, in some persons, by loss of nervous power, while in other persons they seem harmless; but the same differences are seen, and are equally inexplicable, in the case of the muscles. In some persons the same exercise which in other leads to muscular atrophy is followed by the attainment of greater power, and by the growth of the exercised muscles.

"I do not know what lesions ensue in the nerve-fibres when the cord degenerates in the instances referred to above; but the analogy of the muscular atrophy, in which the nerves degenerate with their muscles (though probably only secondarily), makes it probable that the spinal nerves partake of the degeneracy with the cord."

SECT. I—PREMATURE EJACULATION.

Of all the disorders of the sexual organs this is the one that a surgeon most frequently meets with.

Patients complain that semen is emitted so readily, that if they even converse with women, or if they ride on horseback, or walk fast, semen will come away. The friction of the trousers, in some instances, appears sufficient to produce emission; others affirm that ejaculation is attended with scarcely any spasm.[1]

In other instances, erection is hardly complete before emission follows, and then, as the erection immediately ceases, the intended intercourse fails. It is fortunate, considering the disappointment and distress which such a state of things causes, that it is very amenable to treatment.

Hardly any man ever attempted connection for the first time without emission taking place prematurely, sometimes from nervousness, but more frequently, perhaps, from natural impetuosity. This is, as I have said often the case with animals. In most instances the repetition of the act will soon correct this over-rapidity of ejaculation. Whatever the cause, the symptom, if it occurs, should not be neglected or treated lightly; above all, the patient should not be thoughtlessly recommended to repeat his attempts. I have seen some very lamentable cases of complete impotence result from such a course. In addition, however, to the more ordinary causes arising from ignorance, alarm, a bad conscience, or want of power over the will, I would particularly mention another which is not generally appreciated, namely, an excessive irritability of the organs.

A gentleman was sent to me from a midland county suffering from debility of the most marked kind. He was subject to frequent emissions, and the least mental or physical impression produced ejaculation. I desired my patient to uncover the glans; this he was unable to do; he feared either to touch the organ himself, or allow any part to be approached, so great was its sensibility. After several efforts I succeeded in uncovering the glans, and found it coated with hardened, wrinkled, and dry smegma, which was very tenacious. With great care this was washed off, and my patient fainted before I succeeded in removing the secretion. In subsequently passing an instrument, I

---

[1] This rapidity of emission has been likewise noticed, under similar circumstances in animals. Breeders know so well that the first leap which an entire horse takes after being put by for some time will be attended with too rapid ejaculation, that at the end of a few days the mare is again put to the horse.

prising how easily these cases are cured if the irritability is first
of all removed, as in the instance I have mentioned above.
Merely accustoming the glans to the application of air, water, or
lint, will often suffice. Sometimes the passage of a bougie along
the urethra will be necessary, or cauterization may be required.
(See page 291.)

SECT. II.—NON-EMISSION.

The next affection which calls for notice is NON-EMISSION. An
otherwise healthy patient will tell you that he is able to have
connection, the erection is perfect, but no emission follows, and
no pleasurable sensations are felt. I am indisposed to believe
that a patient's sensations can always be depended upon when
the organs have been much abused, for emission may sometimes
take place without his knowledge. There are, however, numberless instances in which emission fails to occur.

Among the causes of this, the most frequent, perhaps, is
stricture, often of old standing. In such a case the mechanical
obstruction prevents the passage of the semen, and it is only
when erection has passed away that the fluid oozes out. In
very severe cases of stricture I believe the semen, if emitted
from the testes, passes back into the bladder instead of forward
along the urethra, and may be noticed in the urine in the form
of a thick, viscous substance. But I would here warn the reader
against mistaking for semen all deposits[1] observed in the urine.
These are of the most miscellaneous and varying composition,
such as mucus from the bladder, the lithates, or the phosphates,
produced by a variety of causes which this is not the place to
inquire into, and which only a medical man can diagnose. True

[1] Patients often require to be warned against considering as semen the
various deposits to be seen, the next morning at the bottom of the vessel into
which they may have made water. If semen is present, it may be noticed
falling to the lower stratum of the urine immediately after micturition. As a
general rule it may be laid down that all deposits falling down when the
urine is cold are not composed of semen. The knowledge of this fact will
give great satisfaction to patients and prevent much misapprehension.

Obstruction, in its early stages, may be suspected when we find the testicles enlarged, painful, and tense, and yet no emissions following sexual intercourse; and also in cases where gonorrhœa has been followed by affections of the testes.

When we bear in mind the frequency of swelled testicle and enlarged inguinal glands, instead of being surprised at the occasional occurrence of these obstructions, we may rather wonder that they do not follow more frequently. Happily, nevertheless, impotence depending upon non-emissions from such causes is rare. Where one testicle or one epididymis or one chord only is affected, the other will carry on all the proper functions. When both chords are blocked up the testes will probably diminish in size until we have hopeless impotence, arising from atrophy of these organs, as well as obstruction of the vasa deferentia. Such cases, I fear, must be considered beyond the reach of our art.

SECT. III.—NOCTURNAL EMISSIONS OR POLLUTIONS. WET DREAMS.

Instead of taking place only during connection, emission may occur at night. The surgeon is usually consulted for cases presenting as nearly as possible the following symptoms :—Patients will tell him that, though leading a continent life, they suffer from emissions at night, and that these generally occur during a dream, and that the penis is at the time in a state of erection.

Great alarm is often expressed by patients who suffer in this way; but I believe that such emissions, occurring once in every ten or fourteen days, are in the nature of a safety valve, and are even conducive to health in persons who do not take enough exercise, and live generously. It would, however, be better for the adult to be free even from these; and I feel convinced that in one who has not allowed himself to dwell on sexual thoughts but takes strong bodily exercise, and lives abstemiously, emissions will either not occur, or their occurrence may be looked for only very occasionally. It is when they take place repeatedly, and leave symptoms of prostration, with other ill consequences, that the patient should seek medical advice.

15

spoken of sleep in its most complete or profound form; that is, the state of complete unconsciousness. But with the absence of consciousness of external things there may be a state of mental activity of which we are more or less distinctly cognizant at the time, and of which our subsequent remembrance in the waking state varies greatly in completeness. The chief peculiarity of this state of *dreaming* appears to be that there is an entire suspension of volitional control over the current of thought which flows on automatically, sometimes in a uniform coherent order, but more commonly in a strangely incongruous sequence. The former is most likely to occur when the mind simply takes up the train of thought on which it had been engaged during the waking hours not long previously, and it may even happen that in consequence of the freedom from distraction resulting from the suspension of external influences the reasoning processes may thus be carried on during sleep with unusual vigor and success, and the imagination may develop new and harmonious forms of beauty. The more general fact is, however, that there is an entire want of any ostensible coherence between the ideas which successively present themselves to the consciousness; and yet we are completely unaware of the incongruousness of the combinations which are thus formed. . . . . . It has been argued by some, that all our dreams really take place in the momentary passage between the states of sleeping and waking; but such an idea is not consistent with the fact that the course of a dream may often be traced, by observing the successive changes of expression in the countenance of the dreamer. It seems, however, that those dreams are most distinctly remembered in the waking state, which have passed through the mind during the transitional phase just alluded to; whilst those which occur in a state more allied to somnambulism are more completely isolated from the ordinary consciousness. There is a phase of the dreaming state which is worthy of notice as marking another gradation between this and the vigilant state; that, namely, in which the dreamer has a consciousness that he is dreaming, being aware of the unreality of the images which present themselves before his mind. He may even make a voluntary and successful effort to prolong

still suffers from nocturnal emissions because he dreams he has
had them.

A case now under treatment will illustrate this. A rather
dreamy-looking individual came to me, after having been under
the care of most of the leading physicians and surgeons in London, complaining that he suffered severely from nocturnal emissions. He was cauterized and recovered his health; he admitted
he had never felt better, and, but for the emissions, would consider himself quite well. I could find nothing the matter with
him; he had gained flesh, he had regained his former bright look,
but he maintained that he had had emissions sixteen times in
the last month. All that I can say was that his looks did not
correspond with his statements. To convince me, he brought
some of the fluid emitted, but I failed in detecting in this any of
the characteristics of semen. I do not believe this patient
wished to deceive me, but I feel convinced he dreamed that
emissions occurred, and probably what he brought me was prostatic fluid.

Such cases deserve great commiseration, for they frequently
arise from hypochondriasis, that strange psychological phenomenon which has often puzzled me as well as other surgeons.
Where it is present it often retards convalescence, as the invalid
cannot bring himself to believe that he is recovering his health
and vigor as long as he thinks himself subject to nightly wet
dreams.

There is a popular belief existing that it is dangerous to
attempt to check emissions. This is as true and as false at the
same time as many popular notions are. It *is* undoubtedly dangerous mechanically to prevent ejaculation, as for instance by
pressure in the perinæum, or by the pressure of a chord tied
around the penis, for in these cases the semen is merely forced
back into the bladder, but not prevented passing from the vesiculæ seminales.

It is dangerous for a man to excite himself, or to allow his
sexual feelings to be excited frequently, and by his will habitually to attempt to check emission; but it is not dangerous, nor is
it attended with any ill consequences, so to train the will that

sions; if they occur one night they are likely to occur the next, and the next. The secret of success is to *break the habit*. The sooner this can be effected the better, and it should be done before the habit becomes imprinted on the system.

It is a fact so generally known that the reader need scarcely be more than reminded of it, that one nocturnal emission in a reduced constitution often weakens the subject of it much more than does connection repeated several times the same night by a healthy person. It is, moreover, a well-ascertained fact, that erotic dreams attended with pleasure leave less weakness than when emissions occur without the knowledge of the dreamer. Explain this as we may, the fact is undoubted; but it is no more to be wondered at than that persons will undergo great exertions and perform extraordinary feats when inspired by hope, and confident of success. We may say such results depend upon nervous influence—others call it courage. It is said that persons so situated have a good tone of the system; that reaction takes place readily. Doubtless the brain or spinal chord has a great influence on the results we are describing, as well as in supporting the loss of semen which some constitutions have the power of renewing much more readily than others.

PREVENTIVE TREATMENT.—In strong robust young men the surgeon need not take much notice of emissions coming on once a week, but recommend the patient to avoid suppers, to abstain from tea, coffee, and tobacco, and to lie on hair or spring mattresses, instead of feather beds, and with only a moderate quantity of clothing.

I recommend my patients to drink no fluid after dinner, supposing that meal to be taken at 6 or 7 o'clock. This and regular evacuation of the bladder at bedtime, will singularly assist the treatment. A very little fluid will be sufficient to relieve any great thirst that may occur in the evening, but the rule should be, avoid drinking after 8 o'clock.

The sufferer should be told that emission usually takes place in heavy sleepers, and the best way of preventing this intense drowsiness in the morning is not to load the stomach over night with all sorts of indigestible and miscellaneous food. Care should

cases to take a voyage on board ship, and keep the watches with the sailor, which allow of taking only four hours' sleep at a time, in the belief that this interruption of rest would break through the almost inveterate habit; but it is difficult in these, the worst forms, to induce the patient to take any trouble to cure himself; he wishes to rely on medicine, and will not give himself the trouble to act independently.

Another very valuable suggestion is to desire the patient to practice the habit of waking early in the morning, turning out of bed, and emptying the bladder. It is in the early morning, when the bladder is full, that emissions and erections take place. In such cases, if a patient rises at 5 or 6, and goes to bed early, he may altogether avoid emissions.

I believe this precaution of keeping the bladder empty at night to be more important than almost anything else in the simpler cases, and that it will be usually successful. I have known an enema of half-a-pint of cold water, used at bedtime, to work well where other means have not produced satisfactory results. It has been said that sleeping between the blankets will prevent emissions, but I cannot say that I have any experience as to this remedy. Tying a towel round the waist, so as to bring a hard knot opposite the spine, will, by preventing the patient from lying on his back, often prevent emissions at night. It is doubtless quite true that the close observer of his own symptoms finds himself generally lying on his back when the emission takes place, but it is equally certain that emissions may occur when the patient lies on his side, as in the following case. One of my most intelligent patients notices that, on suddenly waking on the occurrence of an emission, he finds himself lying on his left side, his legs and knees firmly drawn up against the abdomen, and the erect penis prevented from gaining its natural position by the thighs. Trousseau, in the "Gazette des Hôpitaux," Mai 15, 1856, recommends an instrument to pass up the rectum to press on the vesiculæ, and mechanically prevent the emissions. I have tried the plan on one or two patients, but was obliged to leave it off, as I found that it produced considerable irritation; and even if such clumsy contrivances answered, it

1790. This author says, that since to break the habit is the first object, it is as well to go to the root of it at once, and accordingly recommends the following plan. I have met with one instance in which its manful adoption was attended with perfect success. "An Italian gentleman, of very high station and character, consulted me for quite a different affection; but in order to put me in possession of all the facts in reference to his state of health, he related his history. He had been inconvenienced five years before with frequent emissions, which totally unnerved him. He determined resolutely, that the very instant the image of a woman or any libidinous idea presented itself to his imagination, *he would wake;* and to insure his doing so, dwelt in his thoughts on his resolution for a long time before going to sleep. The remedy, applied by a vigorous will, had the most happy results. The idea, the remembrance of its being a *danger,* and the determination to wake, closely united the evening before, was never dissociated even in sleep, and he awoke in time; and this reiterated precaution repeated during some evenings absolutely cured the complaint."[1]

This plan is founded on such true physiological grounds, that I feel convinced it must succeed in a great variety of cases. To carry it out, however, requires great firmness and resolution, and it will succeed only with those who have habitually exercised self-control.[2]

---

[1] "L'Onanism," p. 241.

[2] A letter I received on this subject some time ago from a very distinguished provincial physician is interesting, and corroborates the above statement as to the possibility of schooling the will so as to awake in time to prevent emission.

"I had no such success," he says, "as to satisfy myself (in overcoming the tendency to emission during sleep), until I adopted the plan of being lightly clad in bed (on a mattress). When not in London studying, I never lay with more than a single sheet on the bed in summer, and a sheet and coverlet in winter, and one blanket extra during keen frosts. Even with this the abomination used to come on about once a month. Indulgence in wine or ale always made the erection more troublesome; but brandy invariably was followed by emission during sleep, without a dream. . . . . . From what a medical friend told me that he had accomplished, I have learned so to school my mind during sleep, that I awake in time to prevent a catastrophe. The

CURATIVE TREATMENT.—When a patient consults me, suffering from the severer form of the complaint, I almost invariably discover, on passing a bougie, an excessive degree of sensibility along the canal. This local cause reacts easily during sleep on the brain, which by reflex action brings on spasm, and hence the frequent emission, which is, as stated at page 234, more or less under the influence of the will. In many instances the passage of an instrument once or twice a week will suffice to remove the morbid irritability, particularly if the treatment be accompanied with some slight stringent injection. It is singular to note the success of this treatment in cases that have resisted all other means previously adopted, such as tonics, &c., and when the surgeon has omitted to accompany his tonics with any local examination.

When, however, this fails, and I admit it occasionally does, I generally have recourse to cauterization, and I find that few cases fail to yield to this treatment, which is attended with little or no pain when performed by a competent surgeon. Cauterization gives the permanent relief that nothing else often will, and I have never yet had cause to regret using it. Those who decry the above methods of treatment cannot, I venture to think, have employed them properly, for both theory and actual practice point them out, in my opinion, as the best means of checking the tendency. As soon as the excessive morbid sensibility of the canal of the urethra has disappeared, the will can assert its force, and then, if the after treatment recommended at page 77 be followed, I am convinced that the health will rally, and it is often surprising to see how the whole physical condition of the patient will improve.

transition from the apparent reality of the dream to the consciousness that the scene is a dream which I must awake from, is very curious. The only occasions when I now suffer are after great fatigue, which involves a profound dreamless sleep. . . . . I do not know whether such things are common, but my father told me that he was very much troubled with wet dreams after he was sixty years of age, sexual desire and connection had ceased and did not return, yet the amount of the discharge was large and weakened him considerably.　　　　　　　　　　I am,

　　　　　　　　　　　　　　　　Yours, very sincerely,

W. ACTON, Esq.　　　　　　　　　　　　　　　——.

Successful as I have generally found this treatment, I must admit that even cauterization will not, in every instance, affect a cure. Every now and then I meet with exceptional cases where the irritation is not confined in the urethra; but either from neglect or from some strong hereditary tendency the habit has already, before any medical aid has been sought, had too serious an influence on the brain or spinal chord to be thus overcome. Instances like these are the rare exceptions, and belong rather to the class of mental diseases, for the discussion of which this is not the place.

In the more severe cases of nocturnal emissions by prescribing opiate enemata in the proportion of sixty or eighty drops of Liq. Opii sedativ. to an ounce and a half of fluid before going to bed, and following the plan recommended at page 236, a cure may generally be effected. In addition to the medical treatment, the patient should be advised to seek cheerful society, but at first to shun association with females. I need hardly add the obvious advice that he should, above all things, break off an acquaintance he may have formed with immodest women. His reading should consist of the light literature of the day, and strict injunctions should be given to abstain from the perusal of any book containing allusion to the subject of his complaint, or any work which would be likely to produce erotic ideas. I frequently have under my care persons who have brought themselves to the last stage of hypochondriacism by reading those pseudo-medical works so generally advertised in the daily papers.

SECT. IV.—DIURNAL POLLUTIONS OR EMISSIONS.

These terms properly include any emission of semen, voluntary or involuntary, during the waking hours. The emission is not necessarily preceded by erection, or attended with pleasure.

In the strictly continent man in good health, who follows the rules of healthy and chaste living, little or no secretion from the urethra will be noticed.

We must, therefore, consider as abnormal all moisture or discharges which the patient notices during the day, and the sufferer who has read in quack books of the exaggerated consequences of these affections, particularly if, as often occurs, he happen to be of a hypochondriacal disposition, will endure great anxiety as to the results. I propose making a few remarks upon these discharges.

I have already stated that, occurring during the day, they are abnormal, and betoken an unimpaired state of health; but at the same time, an occasional loss of even a teaspoonful of secretion will not alone bespeak disorder of the function. It is the repeated leakage, so to speak, that betokens a relaxed patulous condition of the sexual apparatus. I admit that great exaggeration has been indulged in upon the subject, but those who are equally blameable who assert that the symptoms of debility, exhaustion, and impotence, cannot ever depend upon the loss of a little semen. In practice, we find this escape of semen once or twice a day, or every time a patient makes water—goes to the water-closet,—or suffers from sexual excitement,—is attended with a train of symptoms which have a very prejudicial effect on the constitution of a large number of susceptible adults.

It is very easy for any writer to ridicule the idea that the escape of a little fluid should be attended with such serious nervous depression. We must recollect that we are speaking of the loss of semen in an already exhausted individual. No one who has seen much practice can deny the statements of such patients, that one nocturnal emission will debilitate such sufferers for a week; then why, I would ask, disbelieve that one diurnal emission does not produce a similar effect on the already exhausted sufferer? And often such patients will tell you that these losses occur several times a day.

I am ready to admit, however, that the hypochondriacal may exaggerate the influence of these losses, and that possibly what they suffer from may depend upon what they imagine they suffer. But whilst taking into consideration all these circumstances, facts are repeated too often not to satisfy me that a series of well-marked symptoms, namely, those of exhaustive nervous power, attend and follow those diurnal losses. Indeed, they require very accurate diagnosis and appropriate treatment.

If, then, we come to the conclusion that in the daytime emissions occur which give rise to a train of very distressing symptoms, the first question we have to discuss is as to what they consist of. I would lay it down as a rule that these discharges are not necessarily composed of semen. I am rather disposed to believe that in the majority of cases the exuding fluid is more frequently composed of those other secretions which mix with the semen previous to its ejaculation, such as the fluid coming from the vesiculæ seminales and the prostate gland. I am, however, equally certain that in a large number of other cases semen does form a part of the emitted discharge, and when this is the fact must be considered in determining the line of treatment.

When any such secretion is observed to proceed from the meatus of the urethra, the immediately exciting cause is generally one of the following three—*sexual excitement, defecation,* or *micturition.*

DISCHARGES ARISING FROM SEXUAL EXCITEMENT.—In one sense all discharges of this kind take their rise from sexual excitement, for neither by common observation or the microscope can we detect fluid of any kind habitually coming from the urethra at any moment, unless the patient has been subject to more or less sexual excitement. And consequently in a state of health there can be no leakage (so to speak) of semen from the system. Under the influence, however, of sexual desire, a tenacious, transparent fluid frequently oozes from the meatus. Nervous persons pay great attention to this, and will tell their medical adviser a variety of circumstances that they have noticed attending it, and describe the qualities of the discharge with painful minuteness.

Instead of viewing this as an abnormal symptom, it would be very surprising if, under excitement, some such discharge did not occur. If it betokens anything, it is a sign that the patient is potent, as the non-emission of a small quantity of fluid under excitement usually betokens a want of power.

If, however, under very slight excitement—friction of the trousers, &c.—a large quantity of fluid comes away, say a tea-

the morning, or brown bread instead of white with meals, will frequently give great relief. Another very good plan is to commence breakfast with a saucerful of oatmeal porridge.[1]

DISCHARGE DURING MICTURITION.—In a perfectly healthy individual, who has not been subject to sexual excitement, the urine ought to be passed clear to the end, the last drops being as transparent as the first. If, however, sexual excitement has been indulged in, the first as well as the last drops of urine may be somewhat thick, and, if collected and examined under the microscope, traces of spermatozoa may be discovered in them. Such an occasional slight discharge is not what should be stigmatized as a diurnal pollution. In cases, however, where the least amount of straining to make water, or indeed very slight effort, invariably causes a certain quantity of thick fluid to exude after the last drops of urine have been expelled, and when the microscope shows that this fluid contains spermatozoa, and the general health is noticed to suffer from its abundant expenditure, the medical man should be at once applied to.

I am daily convinced that a very considerable proportion of that class of persons who are constantly ailing rather than ill, whose health is impaired, whose spirits are low, and who derive no benefit from tonics, change of air or doctors, are often suffering loss of semen, brought about by marital or other sexual excesses, or in one or more of the ways just specified. I have more than once alluded to the fact that loss of semen (in whatever way

---

[1] As many cooks do not understand how to make the Scotch dish, I append the following directions from Tegetmeier:—"Strew oatmeal with one hand into a vessel of boiling water (to which salt has been previously added), so gradually that it does not become lumpy, stirring the mixture the whole time with the other. After the requisite quantity has been stirred in—namely, about two large handfuls of coarse oatmeal to a quart of boiling water—the whole should be allowed to stand by the side of the fire, so as to simmer gently for twenty-five or thirty minutes. During this time it thickens considerably. As thus prepared it is usually eaten with the addition of milk. There are only a few places in London where a fresh supply can be depended on; that which has been three months in a baker's drawer is to be avoided. Bartrop's in Holborn, and Simpson's, in Skinner Street, Euston Road, I know both to sell good fresh meal at a reasonable price per stone, and doubtless many others do the same.

16

rections in the fluid, just as so many eels would do, by means of their tails, overcoming obstacles in the current, avoiding obstructions, and in fact possessing and exhibiting the power of locomotion to the fullest extent.   Little by little, however, their movements diminish in rapidity and energy.   This depends on two causes—1st, by the actual diminution of the vitality of the spermatozoa themselves; and, 2d, by the condensation of the liquid in which they exist, and which evaporates.   Their progression becomes more difficult, soon they only oscillate, and it seems as if they were held in consequence of their tails becoming fixed in the viscous fluid.   They cease to move, and, in fact, die.   I have, however, seen the movements of these zoosperms last for hours, even days, provided care be taken to protect the fluid in which they are, from evaporation and from cold."—*Cours de Microscopie.*

Such appearances as the above are quite sufficient to distinguish semen from all other fluids under the microscope.   But I need scarcely say that this way of distinguishing semen avails little when it is passed in the urine.   As soon as the spermatozoa become mixed with that fluid, they die and are not to be looked for in the fluid, but are only to be discovered at the bottom of the vessel.   Their discovery under these circumstances is not so easy as Donné's account would lead us to suppose.

To the naked eye I know of no means by which one secretion coming from the urethra can be distinguished from another. Even when diffused in the urine, semen presents no particular appearances; and we cannot distinguish it from the mucus that is often suspended in the urine in the form of a cloud, entangling sometimes epithelial scales, and at other times semen.

PROGNOSIS.—"Diurnal pollutions," Lallemand says, " are (other things being equal) much more difficult to cure than nocturnal emissions; and seminal emissions which attend the simple passage of the urine are more serious and more obstinate than those which take place during the effort of straining in defecation.   In a word, experience proves that the severity of spermatorrhœa is proportioned to the ease with which it takes place, and common sense would predict such a result." (Vol. i, p. 627.)

veloped in the interior of cells, or vesicles of evolution, such as are visible in the seminal fluid in various stages of production (figs. F, G, H, I), and have been known under the head of seminal granules.

"These appear to have been themselves formed within parent cells, which are probably to be regarded as the epithelial cells of the tubuli seminiferi, constituting, like the analogous cells of other glans, the essential elements of the spermatic apparatus. These parent cells are sometimes observed to contain but a single vesicle of evolution, as shown at D; but more commonly from three to seven are seen within them, as in E.

"When the vesicle is completely matured it bursts, and gives exit to the contained spermatozoa. The spermatozoa are not normally found free in the tubuli seminiferi, although they may be there so far advanced in development, that the addition of water liberates them by occasioning the rupture of their envelopes. In the rete testis and vasa efferentia the spermatozoa are very commonly found lying in bundles within the parent cells, the vesicles of evolution having disappeared; and they are usually set free completely by the time that they reach the epididymis, though still frequently associated in bundles. The earlier phases are occasionally met with, however, even in the vas deferens."[1]

That the essential elements of the spermatic fluid are the spermatozoa, may be reasonably inferred from several considerations. There are some cases in which the liquor seminis is altogether absent, so that they constitute the sole element of the semen; but they are never wanting in the semen of animals capable of procreation, though they are absent, or imperfectly developed, in that of hybrids which are nearly or entirely sterile. Moreover, it may be considered as certain that the absolute contact of the spermatozoa with the ovum is requisite for its fecundation. This appears from the fact that, if the spermatozoa be carefully removed from the liquor seminis by filtration, the latter is entirely destitute of fertilizing power. Hence the presence of the liquor seminis must be considered as merely incidental, and

[1] " Human Physiology.' p. 79?, fifth edition.

as answering some secondary purpose either in the development or in the conveyance of the spermatozoa.

Müller says—"Not only are spermatozoa absent from the semen of many animals, and particularly of birds—except at the pairing time—but the development is imperfect in hybrid animals, which are generally incapable of reproducing their kind, or at most pair with individuals of one of the unmixed species, and produce forms which then return to the original fixed type. Hebenstreet, Bonnet, and Gleichen, all failed to detect spermatozoa in the semen of the male mule." (Vol. ii, p. 1478.)

SECRETION OF SEMEN.—Carpenter says, in his "Comparative Physiology," p. 533—

"The development of the spermatozoa is, in most cases periodical, man and most of the domesticated races being the only animals in which there is a constant aptitude for procreation. The spermatic organs, which remain for long periods in a state of atrophy, at particular times take on an increased development, and their product is then formed in great abundance."

The secretion of semen takes place slowly in the continent man—so slowly that, in fact, in many instances, I think little or none is formed in healthy adults whose attention is not directed to sexual subjects, and who take a great deal of strong exercise. The same may be said of animals that are not allowed sexual congress.

QUALITY OF THE SEMEN.—Semen, as we have said (p. 209), when first secreted, is not the same elaborated fluid which we find in the *vesiculæ seminales.* "The complete development of the spermatozoa in their full proportion of number is not achieved till the semen has reached, or has for some time lain in, the vesiculæ seminales. Earlier after its first secretion, the semen contains none of these bodies, but granules and round corpuscles (seminal corpuscles), like large nuclei enclosed within the parent cells. Within each of these corpuscles or nuclei a seminal filament is developed by a similar process in nearly all animals. Each corpuscle or nucleus is filled with granular matter; this is gradually converted into a spermatozoid, which is at first coiled up, and in contact with the inner surface of the wall of the corpuscle."—*Kirkes,* 7th edition, p. 735.

a short time, produce enormous quantities with great rapidity, and probably expend most of it as it is secreted. The periodic enlargement of the testes, and the other changes noticed at the rutting season, supply this requirement. The animal system answers wonderfully to these sudden demands. We observe a similar process when nature is called upon for sudden and extraordinary supplies of horn and bone. Bone, we know, grows very slowly under ordinary circumstances; it is often deposited round fractures in less quantities than we wish it; yet such is the lavishness of nature when called upon, that a stag's antlers will be replaced fully in eleven weeks.

The injected preparation made by John Hunter of the testes of animals that have a rutting season, shows how a healthy male may secrete an almost unlimited quantity of semen for a short time. It should, moreover, be borne in mind that the animal has two testes, only one of which probably is drained at a time, and a large quantity of semen is probably hoarded up in the testes and vasa deferentia.

THE QUANTITY OF SEMEN ACTUALLY EMITTED IN EACH SEXUAL ACT IN MAN amounts, generally, to two teaspoonfuls or one, according as the male has been continent or not. Of course, the whole of this emission does not consist only of pure semen. The secretion, as it leaves the meatus, is a heterogeneous compound. Pittard thus describes it :—"Some dilution, some addition to the volume, seems necessary in order to obtain an efficient injection of the life-giving fluid. And the quantity actually emitted by a man amounts, by all accounts, to two or three drachms. There has, therefore, been an addition somewhere. The prostate has doubtless contributed its share; the tiny glands of Cowper theirs; the urethra has given its mite of mucus, more mucus is waiting in the vagina; and I believe that the vesiculæ are not behind in adding a portion of their ready-formed contribution to the general stock. The spermatozoa, huddled and crowded in countless millions in the vas deferens, are now able to disport themselves at ease in the congenial medium, and the number contained in a few drops of pure semen would be sufficient to people abundantly several drachms of fluid."—*Pittard, in " Cyclop. of Anat. and Phys.," article " Vesiculæ Seminales."*

"Fawns, when cut prior to the formation of any horn—that is, within a week or so after birth—both testes being wholly removed, with a portion of the cord (vas deferens) also, will never bear horns, however long they may live; but if the bodies of the testes only be taken away, the 'knob' (epididymis) being left attached to the cord, the animal will have horns, and renew them annually, the shedding being always rather later in the season, and the velvet covering remaining for a somewhat longer period on their surface than with the entire buck; and, further, they will be more slender in the beam, and more porous in their internal structure. These semi-castrated—if I may so style them—animals will go into rut, but not to the degree which produces emaciation; nor does the great thickening of the neck occur which is so characteristic in the perfect animal during that peculiar season; nor are they capable of procreation. When the adult buck is castrated, the horns are shed shortly afterwards, and renewed; but the persistent periosteum, or 'velvet,' never separates from their surface, and the horns do not again fall, but remain attached during any period the animal may survive. These permanent antlers are often more developed than those produced by entire bucks of equivalent age, which I think may be well accounted for from the fattened state, and the longer influence, from the continued adherence of the vascular integument by which the horns are formed. I may here observe, that circulation continues in the bone or horn after the periosteum has separated, and that, diminishing by degrees, first from the points, the vessels become obliterated, and vitality therefore ceasing, it is cast off."—*Gascoine*, "*On Castration of the Cervidæ;*" "*Proceedings of the Zoolog. Soc.*" *June*, 1856, p. 156.

I have attempted to settle the question of the influence of semen on the system, by inquiries amongst those who have the largest opportunity of studying the subject amongst entire as well as gelded animals, with relation to the enduring qualities in males and females, and this is the information I have arrived at.

There can be no doubt that entire horses are capable of undergoing more work than geldings. It is a saying in Norfolk, that a stallion is equal in draught to one gelding and a half. One such horse is often kept on a farm, and works a certain number of months in the year when not required for that purpose the farmer then puts by, and receives thirty or forty pounds for his mounting services. Such entire horses are not, however always tractable, which is the reason we do not employ them more frequently in England. And the correctness of this opinion has been corroborated by one of the best and boldest riders in England, who tells me he has seen and ridden entire horses, but they soon shut up in the hunting field; they grow sulky and refuse to go. He says on this score they are objectionable; and he gives a stallion a wide berth, as they bite occasionally, and are very vicious. Besides, their tempers are generally uncertain. Although their endurance might be good, it would be rather in draught, he should think, that they might be used. Experience has taught him that they are not adapted for hunting, although they may do for hacks; and here often the same bad temper interferes. He has ridden good geldings as well as good mares, and cannot say which he prefers.

At Tattersall's a gelding is always worth, *cæteris paribus*, £5 more than a mare; this is probably because a mare is liable to kick at the time of horsing. I myself object to drive mares on this score, as no one can be sure of their tempers at these moments.

I was talking the other day to the manager of a large cab company, and remarking on the number of mares the company possesses. "Yes," said he, "geldings, we find are unequal to do the thirty miles a day we expect out of our Hansom cab mares, and we purchase only this description of animal, as suited to our work."

Any one who has travelled much in France must be aware of the fact that stallions are used by preference for all draught purposes; and by means of hard work, and driving in teams together they are made very gentle, even although they are well fed and in excellent condition.

PART II.

DISORDERS AFFECTING THE SEMEN.

WE have now to consider the abnormal and unhealthy conditions which, by influencing the semen, may interfere with the due performance of the sexual act.

SECT. I.—INFECUNDITY—UNFRUITFULNESS—BARRENNESS.

Though the terms are often used loosely as synonymous—"want of power to produce its like" (Barclay)—*unfruitfulness (infécundité)* is not impotence. A man may be unable to beget children, and yet not be impotent, though an impotent man is, of course, unable to beget children.

This state may last a short time, or it may be permanent. Rest may give the semen time to become perfect, or ripen, and the spermatozoa will appear and become mature. Stricture, again, as we have seen, may make a man practically sterile, and so may other affections of the testes or generative organs. Not that infecundity—meaning by that term the lack of children—necessarily rests with the man alone. The cause of non-impregnation may be wholly or partially in the female.

INFECUNDITY IN THE MALE.—Science is very deficient in any accurate examination of the state of the seminal secretions. It is a field still open to the examination of strict observers, and would amply repay the trouble.

Dr. Davy, Assistant-Inspector of Army Hospitals, at the General Military Hospital at Fort Pitt, published in 1858, in the "Edinburgh Medical and Surgical Journal" for July, vol. xl, page 1, a very interesting examination of twenty post-mortem appearances of men who, dying of various diseases, were examined by him,

From this paper I have condensed the following table. The details are reported at great length, as well as the causes of death; the post-mortem appearances, not only of the organs generally, but a minute examination of the secretions found in

the vesiculæ seminales, as well as the microscopical character of
their contents, are given.

No. in Mono-graph.	Age.	Condition of Vesiculæ Seminales.	Condition of Vasa Deferentia.	Examined hours after death.
4	20	Slightly viscid; brown tint	Starchy	11
10	20	Starchy, and gelatinous	Few animalcules; not brown	4
11	27	Partly thick, and partly thin secretion	——	10
14	27	Few spermatozoa, but globules	Healthy, with few spermatic animalcules	32
15	27	Gelatinous; well-formed animalcules	No distinct animalcules, globules	22
13	29	Gelatinous, thick, globules	No fluid in	3
1	30	Similar to that in vasa def.	Numerous animalcules in active motion	6 and 48
17	31	Fluid thick at fundus, in the interior fluid	Globules and fragments	27
5	32	Fluid opaque, purulent	Cream or purulent appearance	16
19	30	Mucilaginous; animalcules numerous	Cream-like globules	22
8	32	Purulent; animalcules abundant	Few animalcules	32
9	33	Small in quantity, brown, opaque	Dilute, purulent — animalcules few	15
12	33	Small in quantity; no animalcules	Small particles; large globules	26
16	33	Globules; no animalcules	Minute globules; no animalcules	6 and 36
6	39	Showed no animalcules; no globules	Purely purulent, with globules; no animalcules	2
3	39	Gelatinous; no animalcules or globules	Of a cream or purulent color; no animalcules	6
20	41	Mucilaginous; many animalcules	Particles, but no animalcules	38 and 58
7	42	Slightly opaque; abundant animalcules	A few animalcules	37
18	49	Animalcules abundant, dead in seventeen hours	Abundant animalcules, lively ten hours	10 and 17
2	57	Abundant vestiges of animalcules; few distinct	Purulent; animalcules abundant, dead	5

The object-glass used was one of one-eighth inch focal distance,
constructed by Moss.

It would appear from the above examination that there is but
little difference in the *microscopic* character of the fluid found in
the vasa deferentia and in the vesiculæ seminales.

In the vasa the *quantity* is smaller, and appears to be in transition from the testes, where it was secreted, into the vesiculæ, where it is retained, and mixed with other secretions.

The fluid found in the vasa deferentia is generally creamy or purulent looking, and is liquid and small in quantity. That found in the vesiculæ is more abundant, of a brownish color—the brown tint increasing after death—and is occasionally tinged with blood. This last, however, may depend upon post-mortem appearances. The two vesiculæ may differ in the quantity of fluid they contain. One may be empty, the other more or less distended.

In consistence the fluid in the vesiculæ varies, being sometimes thin like starch, but more frequently thick, viscid, and gelatinous. After standing a few hours it separates into two parts; the one which subsides being opaque, while the other is transparent; the latter is copiously precipitable by alcohol, and becomes almost gelatinous.

From the above table it appears that the *spermatozoa*, or spermatic animalcules were found equally in the vesiculæ seminales and in the vasa. It is curious to remark that, in all the cases in which spermatozoa were found in the *vasa deferentia*, similar animalcules were noticed in the *vesiculæ seminales*. In cases in which the body was examined a few hours after death the spermatozoa were found alive, and moving actively, while in a few hours later they were motionless and dead, and warmth had no effect in reanimating them. In some cases the animalcules were not perfect, portions only of imperfect spermatozoa being found. In other cases no animalcules could be discovered either in the vasa deferentia or vesiculæ; they were replaced by large or minute globules, small particles, or fragments. The age of the individual appeared to have little to do with this condition of the spermatozoa, or indeed with their presence, numbers, or total absence. It is curious further to remark that, although spermatozoa were found frequently in the vesiculæ and vasa deferentia, they were only found twice in the testes. The fluid expressed from the testes was transparent, generally contained globules nearly equal in diameter to the blood-corpuscles, and

17

gotten that idiosyncracies exist in all animals. A male and female may be perfectly potent and fertile, and yet be unable to breed together. In fact, the semen of one male, from some hidden cause, will not impregnate a particular female, though it will others. A similar phenomenon occurs also in the vegetable world.

In Mr. Darwin's book on the "Origin of Species," there are some curious experiments mentioned bearing on this question. "Thus one tree will not take (be grafted) on another, apparently from differences in their rate of growth, in the hardness of the wood, in the period of the flow, or nature of their sap. On the contrary, great diversity in these very particulars, and even in more important ones, are not infallible tests. One may be woody and the other herbaceous—one evergreen and the other deciduous—one the native of a hot climate, the other of a cold one—and the grafts from one on the other may succeed. The pear can be grafted far more readily on the quince, which is ranked as a distinct genus, than on the apple, which is a member of the same genus. Even different varieties of the pear take with different degrees of facility on the quince; so do different varieties of the apricot and peach on certain varieties of the plum." (p. 261.)

"Sterility may be produced by the attempt to cross between very different races. An embryo may be developed to a considerable extent, but the mother's system never recovers the disturbance caused by the attempt to unite two organizations so widely unlike. This often happens, according to Mr. Hewitt, in attempts to cross among gallinaceous birds." (p. 264.)

That one horse will fail to impregnate a mare, while she will prove in foal by another, is well known to breeders. During the season of 1864, I sent a mare several times to be served by a particular horse, but without success, while, on being put to another, she was immediately impregnated. I observed the same in the case of a very celebrated high-bred short-horned bull, in my own neighborhood, which, although he mounted cows, did not impregnate them. These and other anomalies deserve the consideration and close observation of all breeders of valuable stock.

would often be less inducement for them thus to demean themselves were greater pains taken to render their homes agreeable, and especially by providing that they shall learn in the domestic circle to enjoy the society of modest women.

Similar consequences, only in a modified way, follow long engagements, and are witnessed also in the many instances where worthless wordly women trifle with serious men's affections to jilt them in the long run.

These consequences are not confined to single life. I remember one very painful case in which the patient's wife—to whom he was passionately attached—was the real cause of serious illness in her husband, by obdurately refusing to allow marital intercourse, for fear of having any more children (she had several), although she otherwise kept up the semblance of familiarity and affection, and thus added very greatly to his suffering.

Few medical men would, however, venture to suggest such a cause for the general ill-health and sexual debility they meet with, but I am sure such cases are not unfrequent ; and where the excitement is allowed to continue, all the remedies of the Pharmacopœia will avail nothing, and in the more severe cases, I fear that even subsequent abstinence from all causes of excitement will not ensure a cure. I have every reason to believe that if the consentaneous performance of what constitutes the sexual act be repeatedly disturbed, the best medical treatment is not always efficacious in restoring sexual power.

These ailments, I repeat, are not confined to the young. There are old men who marry young wives, and who pay the penalty by becoming martyrs to paralysis, softening of the brain, and drivelling idiocy. Such unions as these, whether in the young or old, are certain sooner or later to do mischief. I am daily made cognizant that many cases of the most intractable forms of impotence I have to treat arise from similar causes. In the first place, these indulgences—which are thought so harmless—produce local mischief in the reproductive organs. Among the principal and primary evils they cause, is the weakening of that consentaneous actions which should connect the excitement of the organs and the complete performance of the sexual act. In the next stage, the excited nervous system, if it does not receive that shock which we have seen attends ejaculation, suffers a longer and more severe strain, lasting often days or nights, and one which is repeated over and over again. In fact, the non-occurrence of emission after sexual excitement permits for a time the repetition of the excitement; but ultimately a collapse takes place from which it is very difficult to rally a patient. The consequences are, that when after the preliminary excitement has occurred, and the control of the will shall have been able to prevent emission, the patient will very probably find that when he wishes it, emission will not follow erection. These practices, unnatural in the highest degree, cannot be carried on with impunity. Nature is sure, sooner or later, to inflict a severe retaliation.

I cannot bring to a close this important chapter without directing the attention of the profession to the dangers that married couples incur *in defrauding nature*. A writer in the "Lancet" has lately stigmatized the practice as CONJUGAL ONANISM, and a Mr. Bergeret has in a French work entitled "Des Fraudes dans l'accomplissement des fonctiones generatrices," given a very succinct account of how it is that French parents determine (and carry out) that they shall only have one, or at most two children. M. Bergeret mentions that this practice of limiting the family is not confined to the poor; the system also holds good among the upper classes in France. In a discussion which took place a few years ago in the French Academy, it was publicly admitted that the arrest in the progressive augmentation of the population in France did virtually depend upon the means the nation took to check its increase by *fraude génésiques*.

I am far from attributing, with the author of this treatise, so many of the local ill consequences which he traces in the female to the means pursued. On the contrary, I am fully convinced that the many ailments which M. Bergeret considers to follow the practices followed in France attend—although, perhaps, in a less degree—married life in England, where, I am happy to say, the practices are hardly known, and still less frequently practised. Still I raise a warning voice against either married or unmarried persons giving themselves up to ungratified sexual excitement.

SECT. III.—SEXUAL SUFFERING IN THE MARRIED.

In speaking of continence (page 56), I admitted the difficulties some young men experienced in maintaining it, and I furnished some important evidence proving that a strong will, plenty of exercise, and surgical supervision, would enable a man to control his sexual appetites. In the present section I propose devoting a few pages to the sexual suffering in the married—a subject which has not met with that consideration from medical men which it deserves.

It often occurs that married men come to me with sad complaints of the intense suffering they have to undergo. I saw such a patient to-day. He was a man of strong sexual disposition, married, and the father of several children. In consequence of the rapidity with which his wife (a delicate woman) had brought him a family, she had been suffering severely from uterine disease, for which she was then under treatment, and the medical attendant had recommended separate beds and abstinence from all sexual relations. This patient assures me that no one could imagine what torments he has undergone, warmly attached as he is to a loving, educated, and beautiful wife, yet debarred from all the most cherished advantages of a married man. "What could I recommend?" was his inquiry.

Let me cite another instance. Such a man as the above came to me with a budget of grievances. Married to a woman of strong animal instincts she had proved unfaithful to him, and an action for divorce was about being brought by my patient against the lady. *En attendant* my married patient was the subject of most acute sexual suffering, without any immediate chance of becoming legally separated from a woman who, although his wife, had ceased to be a wife to him; yet society had decreed that he must bear his hard lot, without any chance of being

speedily released from the most acute sexual suffering. Moving
in the best and most fashionable society, much admired and sym-
pathized with by the sex, he assured me that no one could form
any idea of the sufferings or temptations he had hourly to undergo; yet he was chained to this torment, and his every action
watched by the most vigilant social police that the friends of the
wife could call to their aid.

I regret to say that I can but offer my sympathy in such cases
as these, but I have promised my patients to bring their grievances before my profession, and I truly think their sufferings deserve consideration.   To persons who are thus situated my remarks on continence are of value; I admit that the distress I
have attempted to depict is not sensational, but how law or equity
can assist the sufferer I am unable to decide.   As a surgeon, I
have no hesitation in saying that a man of strong sexual disposition must make many sacrifices.   He must eschew much
agreeable female society, he should abstain from the indulgences
of the table, and he must take more exercise than the indolent
are disposed to adopt.   The profession can offer him little assistance and but little benefit, unless he be indeed endowed with a
strong will—an aid to the treatment often found wanting in
strongly-developed animal natures.   Is it surprising, then, that
so many who, under more favorable auspices, would have made
the best of husbands, fall victims to a vicious mode of living, and
seek in fornication some alleviation of their sexual sufferings?

These are some of the arcana of social life that are revealed
only to medical men, in the hope (often a vain hope) that they
may be in a position to suggest some mode of relief.

During the last few years, and since the rights of women have
been so much insisted upon, and practically carried out by the
"strongest-minded of the sex," numerous husbands have come
urging me to represent to the tribunals of the country the hard-
ships under which they suffer by being married to women who
regard themselves as martyrs when called upon to fulfil the
duties of a wife.   This spirit of insubordination has become the
more intolerable—the husbands assert—since it has been backed
by the opinions of John Stuart Mill, who in his recent work on

the "Subjection of Women," would induce the sex to believe that they are "but personal body-servants of a despot." Mr. Mill complains that the wife has not even the privilege of the female slave, who he states "has (in Christian countries) an admitted right and is considered under a moral obligation to refuse to her master the last familiarity. Not so the wife; however brutal a tyrant she may be chained to—though she may know that he hates her—though it may be his daily pleasure to torture her, and though she may feel it impossible not to loathe him—he can claim from her and enforce the lowest degradation of a human being, that of being made the instrument of an animal function contrary to her inclinations."

As opposed to these doctrines, I would rather urge the sex to follow the example of those bright, cheerful, and happily constituted women, who, instead of exaggerating their supposed grievances, instinctively, as it were, become the soothers of man's woes, their greatest gratification apparently being to minister to his pleasures, seeing that woman was created for the purpose of being a help-meet to her husband. Doubtless many a medical man can, like myself, recall the bitter confessions of more than one married woman who, in her repentant moments, has acknowledged that want of sympathy and affection on her part has led first to estrangement and subsequently to a permanent separation from a husband whose merits she has learned too late to appreciate.

SECT. IV.—DISAPPOINTMENTS IN LOVE.

Disappointment in love or misplaced affections are frequently attended with most painful sexual consequences, even among men who are not usually thought very susceptible. In October, 1861, I attended a patient who came to me complaining that his health was breaking down, and that (as his medical attendant had told him) he was suffering from loss of semen. It appeared that he had led an almost continent life; and, after having by strenuous exertion attained a position of some eminence, had

ally disappear under the careful administration of these salts and a patient restored to health if he has the will strong enough to abstain from exposing himself to similar trials.

I believe cases similar to the one just related are much more common than is supposed, and I have selected one as a type of the ignorance and carelessness with which young men will injure their health by conduct which a very little knowledge would convince them is dangerous to the last degree. Of course this state of health may arise from other čauses; but the numerous instances in which debility does undoubtedly follow from this cause serve to show that a man cannot with impunity disobey natural laws. Sexual excitement is intended to be followed by sexual gratification, and the pent up feelings both physical and mental will pretty certainly, as I have already said, avenge themselves on both mind and body in a way equally unexpected and destructive.

SECT. V.—PASSING BLOODY SEMEN.

Occasionally patients not only complain of emission taking place at unusual times, but state that the semen is colored red. I have very recently had such a case under my care. It occurred in a married man about fifty, who, as far as I could learn, had committed no excesses: he was surprised one night by an emission, to which he had not been previously subject, and, to his further astonishment, observed that the night-shirt was stained with blood. As soon as he could dress he came to consult me; I could find nothing unusual in his urine, nor could I discover any lesion of the canal. Although this patient was under my care for some days subsequently, no recurrence either of the bloody discharge or the emission took place. In other instances that have come under my notice, I am inclined to think that some mechanical injury must have happened to the penis during sleep, so as slightly to rupture the lining membrane. At any rate I doubted in this particular instance whether the blood was in any way mixed with the semen, except at the very moment of ejaculation.

less been indulged in by many of those who have described the complaint, and this from obvious and infamous motives; but I am convinced, as I have already stated, that many of the most obstinate as well as obscure complaints which the medical man meets with arises from the repeated loss of semen, and I am no less certain that hypochondriasis, the various forms of indigestion, debility, and nervous affection, with loss of sleep, are often only the effects of spermatorrhœa. In such cases the best, and indeed the only treatment, is that which removes the *cause*, and is not confined to combating the symptoms. The best evidence of this cause and effect is, that such radical treatment alone relieves the symptoms when all other remedies have failed.

The condition or ailment which we here characterize as *Spermatorrhœa*, then, as we shall use the word, is a state of enervation produced, at least primarily, by the loss of semen. The term, I admit, has many objections, but its general acceptance would render it inconvenient to alter it or employ any other. The disease, however, has received many other titles. No doubt can exist that the series of symptoms—here spoken of—were well known to the ancients. Hippocrates, for example, describes it thus: " *Tabes dorsalis* proceeds from the spinal cord, it is frequently met with among newly married people and libertines. There is no fever, the appetite is preserved, but the body falls away. If you interrogate the patients, they will tell you that they feel as if ants were crawling down along the spine. In making water or going to stool, they pass much semen. If they have connection the congress is fruitless; they lose semen in bed, whether they are troubled with lascivious dreams or not— they lose it on horseback or in walking. To epitomize, they find their breathing become difficult, they fall into a state of feebleness, and suffer from weight in the head and a singing in the ears. If in this condition they become attacked with a strong fever, they die with cold extremities."

In a great number of individuals, both young and adult, an enervated state of body exists, which the profession, as well as patients when attacked with marked loss of semen, characterized by the somewhat vague term Spermatorrhœa, a complaint (I

inary circumstances the marriage was postponed. He complained of nearly all the symptoms which constitute spermatorrhœa, and was naturally alarmed at his state; this I could and did assure him was temporary. After contrasting the conditions of the continent and incontinent man, I think I succeeded in convincing him that the only danger he had to dread, arose from continuing venereal excess; that, if he remained continent, the temporary result of vigorous mental exertion would pass away, leaving him none the worse; but that the double strain on both the brain and the generative system—against which nature herself appeared to take this means of appealing—would most certainly deteriorate if not ruin both.

I have become more and more convinced of the large proportion of students in all professions who suffer in a similar manner. My usual advice to them, in addition to maintaining strict continence, is to continue their studies, but by no means to neglect regular bodily exercise. Benefit is also derived by abstaining from the use of coffee, tea and tobacco.

In the more nervous cases the occasional passage of a bougie will dull the acute sensibility too often present in these sufferers, and give the patient that control of the will that is most desirable in such afflicting cases.

Masturbation and Venereal excesses.—That these are the chief causes of spermatorrhœa appears sufficiently from the former part of this work, to which I refer the reader for a description of both, and their effects, as well as (p. 152) for a definition of what constitutes excess.

Nevertheless, a large proportion of cases of spermatorrhœa depend upon other causes; and I desire particularly to dwell upon this fact, and to obtain its recognition, inasmuch as the complaint is not always a self-inflicted one, and when this is the case the stigma attached to it may be undeserved.

Nervous affections are often the cause of spermatorrhœa; still I am not prepared to say that these nervous affections themselves may not be consequences of previous masturbation or venereal excesses. It is very difficult in some instances, and especially in

18

the later stages, to determine what relation they bear to the spermatorrhœa, as in the following instance.

In September, 1859, a tall, cadaverous, worn-looking man, called on me, complaining of pain in the head, disordered digestion, impaired intellect, loss of memory, uncertain gait, difficulty of progression, and uncertainty in putting his foot forward. His history was that of many others related in these pages; early excesses, mental distress in consequence—feeble resolves, followed by miserable failures and bitter repentance. Whether his present condition really arose altogether from these causes or from what is vaguely called a nervous affection—chiefly because no cause can be assigned to it—I could not for some time determine. One or two indications which pointed to local irritation of the generative organs still existing, decided me to try the treatment appropriate to a case of undoubted spermatorrhœa. The result proved that my surmise was right, and the nervous affections disappeared with the local symptoms.

Other cases, however, exist which are clearly traceable to nervous affections of hereditary origin. I have for years attended a young man who has suffered, off and on, from some of the most severe symptoms of this malady. He tells me his mother has been a martyr to nervous affections, and his family all more or less labor under various hysterical and nervous disorders. In the male these functional disturbances often assume the form of spermatorrhœa in cases where I am persuaded no vicious habits have been practised. I am not so sure, however, that in married life sexual excesses have not aggravated the symptoms, as reference to Chapter on Marital Excesses, page 148, will show.

Nocturnal emissions, as they induce loss of semen, act as a very frequent exciting cause of spermatorrhœa. (p. 230.)

Marital excesses act exactly in the same way. I need not here repeat what I have said at page 148, further than again to point out that excessive loss of semen from whatever cause will produce the very effects which are usually classed under the general term of spermatorrhœa. (p. 277.)

SYMPTOMS.—True spermatorrhœa, as has been stated, consists not in any one particular symptom, but rather in a train of symptoms which make up the affection. One or two of these, however, are so prominent, and yet are such fertile sources of error that it may be as well to mention them separately. And first,

Loss of Semen.—A patient will come to his medical adviser, stating that he is constantly losing semen, either by day or night, or both. This may be true, and, if true, is a serious thing, but alone it does not constitute spermatorrhœa. In nine cases out of ten, however, the statement is much exaggerated, or only very partially true. The first duty of the surgeon, therefore, is to ascertain the nature of the fluid passed. If the patient make water in a test-tube, and the water is allowed to stand and cool, various deposits may be thrown down, any of which are sufficient to account for his alarm, but none of which need necessarily arise from the presence of semen in the water, thus :—

The urine when first passed may be milky or slightly turbid. This, as I shall presently show, depends upon a deposit of phosphates, which, although a symptom to be attended to and requiring medical interference, depends in no way on semen in the urine.

In other instances, small floating atoms or flocculi may be seen floating in the liquid passed, and which the patient will point to as, in his opinion, presenting undoubted proofs of the affection. These the medical man will be enabled to tell him are nothing but epithelial cells thrown off by the mucous membrane, and are a sign of gleet, which, of course, should be treated; but, happily, spermatorrhœa, is not the affection the patient suffers from.

The suspension of mucus in the urine as it cools will often be pointed out as semen. This—depending upon some slight irritation of the bladder—may be easily distinguished by the medical man from semen.

Again, after the urine has stood some little time, a white floculent matter may be observed deposited at the bottom of the test-tube or suspended in the lower half of the fluid. Instead of becoming white this deposit may be of a brick-red color. The patient may be assured that these deposits are the urates or lithates depending upon indigestion, and a means by which the system throws off superfluous nourishment.

Long streamers or cottony-looking flocculi are now recognized as coming from the prostate or the vesiculæ seminales; the masses of mucus, of all kinds of secretions and the vermicelli-like threads are only broken-down epithelium, or may depend upon a neglected stricture or old gleet, and are all quite independent of the testes and their secretions.

These appearances will be most evident in the morning, particularly when the night has been restless, or after breakfast, when nervous excitement has come on, or the digestion has been impaired. The test-tubes used for the purpose of examining these deposits, I may mention, should be much larger than the ordinary ones, large enough to enable the patient to make water directly into them; the urine, when cold, can be thus accurately examined.

The microscope will dissipate the fear which most of the above appearances raise.

Lastly, and most rarely, the microscope detects the presence in the urine of spermatozoa, dead or alive, but most frequently the former, as urine is fatal to them: and they are to be looked for at the bottom of the tube, where they may be seen mixed with the other secretions above alluded to.

Although this comparatively rare symptom of the constant involuntary loss of semen is one of the symptoms of true spermatorrhœa, it does not by any means follow that, whenever spermatozoa are found in the urine, the patient is suffering from spermatorrhœa; for as we have shown above (see page 236), semen occasionally passes away naturally under certain conditions.

Non-erection or *imperfect erection*, in the opinion of some nervous patients, is sufficient to prove that they have spermatorrhœa, and coupled with other symptoms no doubt can exist that these symptoms require careful investigation; but I must refer my readers to pages 200 and 202 for their fuller consideration.

Lallemand thus describes *other local symptoms:* "If excesses are carried far enough, or last long enough, the excitement augments; and the first symptoms of irritation manifest themselves. Heat in the canal commences, particularly during the act of making water, the urine is more abundant than usual, and the desire to pass it more frequent, accompanied with a tickling which is sometimes agreeable; the meatus is more injected than usual, and the intensity of pleasure is diminished."

In another place he says—" One of the earliest symptoms of spermatorrhœa consists *in a diminution of pleasure* during the act, even before the general health has become deranged." He continues—

"At the same time that the sensation becomes weakened, erections are less complete and prolonged; ejaculation is more rapid; it becomes, in fact, so precipitate, that intromission cannot take place. The act, in regard to its duration, is almost reduced to nothing, and the same may be said of the other phenomena; it consists of a simple *excretion of semen;* we should moreover add that the seminal liquor is little abundant, watery, transparent, without smell, and incapable of fecundation." (Vol. i, p. 623.)

One of the worst features is when, in the words of this author,—

"Little by little, the phenomena of excitement which precede the orgasm diminish, and at last completely disappear; the emission then occurs without dreams, without erection, without pleasure, and even without any particular sensation; in fact, the patients are not aware that emission has taken place except by the stains which they observe on the linen when they awake. At the same time the seminal fluid loses by degrees its consistence, its color, its smell, and resembles most closely mucus or prostatic fluid." (Vol. ii, p. 329.)

The same author remarks, and I quite coincide in his opinion,—

"Every exaggerated evacuation of semen is susceptible of producing similar effects on the economy, in whatever way it may have been produced." Thus masturbation, marital excesses, or licentious habits will produce one and the same effect. Moral-

known as falsetto.   Not only ˚non-development, but repeated loss of semen and abuse of the sexual organs has a perceptible effect in some cases upon the timbre of the voice.

It has not, however, until quite lately been noticed how closely those affections of the throat, so commonly met with in young and continent men, and known generally under the term clergyman's throat, are connected with disorders or disturbances of the sexual organs.

That sexual intercourse has the singular effect of producing dryness of the throat has long been known.   Masturbation often repeated, or profuse nocturnal emissions, have the same effect; and in process of time this symptom, which at first is only temporary, may become permanent.   Of course the throat affection may arise from many other causes, but I have seen it so frequently associated with excesses which have debilitated the reproductive organs, that little doubt exists in my own mind that in the majority it is the *consequence* more or less direct of those excesses, and not merely a casually contemporaneous affection. That this must be so is proved, moreover, by finding the throat-symptom often cured by the treatment adopted to relieve the generative ailments, though they have resisted all other.   When the *fons et origo mali* has been reached, the hoarseness disappears under appropriate treatment with great rapidity.

The following are notes taken down and sent to me by a young clergyman who was a sufferer from the complaint, and had derived no benefit from any treatment of the specific affection till the sexual symptoms had been overcome:

"When I began the practice of masturbation, at the age of 16, I was in the habit of exercising my voice regularly.   The first part in which I felt the bad effects of that habit, was in the organs of articulation.   After the act, the voice wanted tone, and there was a disagreeable feeling about the throat which made speaking a source of no pleasure to me as it had been.   By-and-by, it became painful to speak after the act.   This arose from a feeling as if a morbid matter was being secreted in the throat, so acrid that it sent tears to the eyes when speaking, and would have taken away the breath if not swallowed.   This, however, passed away in a day or two after the act.   In the course of years, when involuntary emissions began to impair the constitution this system became permanent.   The throat always feels very delicate, and there is often such irritability in it, along with this feeling of the secretion of

morbid matter, as to make it impossible to speak without swallowing at every
second or third word. This is felt even in conversation, and there is a great
disinclination to attempt to speak at all. In many instances, in which the
throat has been supposed to give way from other causes, I have known this
to be the real one. May it not be that the general irritation always produced
by the habit referred to, shows itself also in this organ, and more fully in
those who are required habitually to exercise it?"

Another case, of a different kind, may be interesting. A boy,
fifteen years of age, was sent to me by a medical man in the
country for an opinion as to his general state of health. He was
small in stature, pale in face, with large ears, and prominent,
thick lips. I noticed that he spoke thickly, and was very dull
of comprehension. His health, I was told, had been failing for
some time and had not benefited under the ordinary treatment.
The throat was painful, the tonsils swollen, the articulation thick,
and the words uttered with evident difficulty. The expression of
his features irresistibly suggested vice and early sensuality.

On inquiry I found that this youth had been taken from school
as he made no progress and had been petted at home. In reply
to some searching questions, I learnt from the boy that he had
masturbated himself at school three or four times a week for a
long time; that the affection of the throat then became a prominent symptom, and that the condition of the throat was but one
of a series of symptoms, all of which I had no difficulty in refer-
ring at once to the excesses of which he had been guilty. I may
add that, under proper treatment, this unpromising case recovered, and the youth is now able to pursue his studies with advantage, and in the holidays rides well across country.

Irritation of the Genital Organs and Scrotum.—A not less
serious and distressing consequence of masturbation is the local
irritation caused by it. A case which came under my notice in
1862, may serve as an example. Similar ones are by no means
uncommon.

Dr. ———— wished me to see a case of his, a tutor in a family,
who had been for eighteen months suffering severely, and whose
symptoms had resisted all remedies. On examination, I found
the testes large and somewhat pendulous. There were no external
symptoms of mischief to be observed, yet the patient complained

of all sorts of uneasy sensations, weight, pain, and such severe irritation of all the genital organs, as to keep him awake during the greater part of the night, and to render his life a burden to him. I examined his urine, which was normal; I passed an instrument (bulbed bougie) and could detect no particular local irritation of the urethra. The patient, however, acknowledged that he thought his ailments might depend upon masturbation, which he had practised formerly, and even now he had not entirely abandoned, the desire being occasionally so strong as to amount almost to a sort of satyriasis. He had never had connection or even attempted it. He was a freshly-colored man with somewhat sunken eyes. One of his most distressing symptoms was frequent and painful erection, and I advised cauterization as the best treatment under the circumstances.

THE PROGNOSIS OF SPERMATORRHŒA.—We may usually give a very favorable opinion, in case of spermatorrhœa, as to the prospect of a cure if the surgeon be consulted in the early stages of the complaint. Unfortunately, ignorance on the part of the patient regarding the nature of the affection, general stimulants prescribed by some medical man, and the false delicacy of the sufferer often cause much delay and anxiety to the patient.

But, however confident we may be in giving a favorable prognosis relative to the disappearance of special and local symptoms in cases of spermatorrhœa, we must be somewhat cautious, when the nervous system has been once impaired, in promising perfect and speedy restoration of the natural sensations or feelings, or more than a very partial return to the buoyant state of health the patient previously enjoyed. We can guarantee, even in severe cases, a comforable state of existence, but the patient must not expect his countenance will at once lose its haggard expression, or that his broken health will be immediately restored. His nervous system has received a shock from which it takes time to recover. Travel, amusing and intellectual employment, with cheerful society and the comforts of life which easy pecuniary circumstances give, do certainly sometimes effect greater cures than I at first had even dared to prognosticate.

DIAGNOSIS.—The diagnosis of these affections is easy enough

found in the urine at the time it is passed, or which may be discovered after allowing it to stand. In these cases of difficult diagnosis the microscope and chemistry generally enable us to decide on the nature of the secretion. Three rules, however, should never be forgotten, rules which are of equal value to the nervous patient and the medical man.

1st. Spermatozoa or traces of them are always to be found in a seminal discharge. To discover the presence of spermatozoa we should desire the patient, as I have already said, to micturate into a long and narrow tube capable of containing an ounce of fluid, and place it for a few minutes in a test-rack. The spermatozoa, in consequence of their greater specific gravity, will, if present, sink to the bottom of the fluid. If there is much saline matter, it may be dissolved by adding plenty of water and letting the mixture stand, when the spermatozoa will sink as before. Donné asserts that the fluid may even be boiled without destroying them. The same author states that he has discovered spermatozoa in urine several days after it has been passed (Loc. cit., p. 315).

2d. The presence of spermatozoa in urine does not conclusively prove the existence of spermatorrhœa, or even of constant seminal discharge. The effort of difficult micturition, or defecation, the fact of the patient having lately had connection, or even of having undergone sexual excitement, is enough to account for the first subsequent emission of urine containing spermatozoa. A small quantity of semen may have been left in the urethra and pass away with the first stream. It is not then the occasional presence of spermatozoa in the urine, but the habitual escape of semen coupled with general symptoms of debility that constitutes the condition—Spermatorrhœa.

3d. Spermatorrhœa may really exist, though it may be impossible at first to discover spermatozoa in the urine.

Donné gives some interesting particulars of cases of suspected discharge of semen which he has watched for days together without finding any traces of spermatozoa. After several days, perhaps, the discharges all at once were found to contain large quantities of spermatozoa. In one case, during eighteen days the urine was most carefully examined several times a day, and yet on three occasions only could the spermatozoa be detected, and each time the patient was aware that a nocturnal emission had occurred. In other instances all the urine passed during the night may contain spermatozoa, while that passed in the daytime is found to be perfectly free from them (Loc. cit., pp. 329–332).

It frequently happens also that at the time of consulting the surgeon, a patient no longer passes semen, this stage of the complaint having passed by. Consequently, the closest examination fails to detect any spermatozoa in the urine, though the patient is suffering all the consequences of loss of semen, and presents all the other symptoms of spermatorrhœa. What we have to decide is, whether the general and local symptoms (and not one symptom only) are such as indicate what we have here called Spermatorrhœa.

These simple rules and remarks should be carefully studied by patients, who are only too ready to fall into error on this subject, or, still worse, into the hands of quacks, and to suppose, or be persuaded, that all discharges that follow or attend micturition, consists wholly or partially of semen. A very nervous patient, who had lately married, and whose wife was in the family way, came to me complaining of impaired health and of frequent emissions in passing urine, although he occasionally indulged in sexual intercourse. I desired him to make water in my presence, and he did so about two hours after breakfast. As the last glassful of urine came away, the patient called my attention to the so-called semen, and I could scarcely be surprised at his terrors, especially as I knew he had heard and read a great deal of Spermatorrhœa. A thickish fluid, in color and consistence resembling cream, dropped into the glass, and in a few seconds fell to the bottom, the supernatant fluid being more or less transparent. The patient stated that this discharge took place only occasionally, and most frequently after breakfast, and as the subsequent effects were invariably debilitating, he felt no doubt that the secretion was really semen. I was able easily to reassure my patient, and to convince him that his creamy discharge was nothing but a deposit of phosphates, as a little acid poured into the test-tube caused the instantaneous disappearance of the so-called semen.

PATHOLOGY.—Little is known as to the local condition which gives rise to this complaint. I believe that in the earlier phases little or no local change takes place, the affection being functional only.

In the more advanced cases, however, we find an enormously increased sensibility. The mucous membrane is susceptible to both local and general influences to a surprising degree. This irritability leaves no traces after death, and I am not aware that any post mortem examination has ever been made which throws any light on the subject.

In some instances there is, during life, an increased redness and tenderness of the meatus, glans, or urethra, but these symptoms do not necessarily occur.

Of the Urethra.—In the advanced stages, when irritation or inflammation has existed for some time in the genito-urinary systems, or nocturnal or diurnal pollutions have been established, and pain, dysuria, or a frequent desire of passing urine occur, the surgeon will notice—when he introduces an olivary bougie, about the size of No. 8—that for the first three or four inches it passes readily enough ; at this point of the instrument's progress some patients will complain of pain, and as it advances towards the bladder the more susceptible will sometimes accuse you of cutting them with a knife, so acute is the suffering, even when the bougie is passed by one who has a delicate hand. When the instrument reaches the bladder, and is allowed to remain at rest for a few minutes, the pain ceases, and on withdrawing it the suffering is slight, and no blood follows ; a drop or two, however, may sometimes ooze out. In these cases, then, we may naturally suppose (for I have never had an opportunity of verifying my opinion on the dead subject) that we have to deal either with simply a morbid sensibility of the mucous membrane about the verumontanum (see Diagram, p. 286), or else with a granular condition, similar to that observed sometimes on the inner surface of the eyelids, and occasionally in other mucous membranes, as a consequence of chronic inflammation.

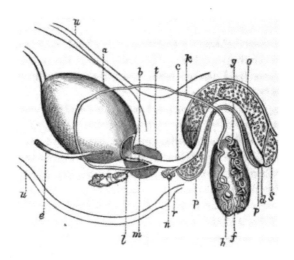

DIAGRAM SHOWING A SIDE VIEW OF THE MALE REPRODUC-
TIVE ORGANS.

Explanation of Figures.

a Bladder.

b Prostatic portion of the urethra laid open, showing the position of the veru-montanum or caput gallinagenis, and how the different canals conveying fluid from the Vesiculæ Seminales and Prostate meet and mix their secretions with that of the semen (proper) coming from the testicles.

c Membranous portion of the urethra.

d Spongy portion of the urethra.

e Right ureter as it enters the bladder.

f Testicles (right).

g Epididymis globus major.

h Epididymis globus minor.

k Vas deferens (right).

l Vesicula seminalis (right).

m Ejaculatory duct.

n Cowper's gland.

o Corpus cavernosum of the penis.

p Bulb of the urethra.

r Corpus spongiosum of the urethra.

s Corpus spongiosum of the glans penis.

t Prostate (bisected).

v Anus.

uu Anterior walls of abdomen, and outline of sacrum.

The reader will see in the above Diagram the relative positions of the reproductive organs most admirably portrayed. I have much pleasure in acknowledging the advantage I have derived from the kind assistance of Mr. Callender, who has corrected the anatomical relations.

Again, there may be stricture of the urethra near the vera-montanum, causing the semen to pass back into the bladder instead of forward along the urethra.

Of the Vesiculæ Seminales.—" The vesiculæ seminales," says Lallemand, " may be dilated and thickened ; they may lose their characteristic irregular, uneven surface, and become firmly adherent to the surrounding structures. Their lining membrane may be covered with lymph, or granular fungoid vegetations. They may be filled with pus or tuberculous matter.

" I have almost always found in the vesiculæ seminales, particularly at the bottom of the depressions, a thick, granular, shining liquid, variable in its aspect, color, and consistence, but resembling pretty thick glue, and more or less transparent. Under a power strong enough to observe the spermatozoa, the particles[1] (grumeaux) of this secretion appear somewhat irregular in size, more or less opaque, and of a constant shape. These are evidently the products of the internal membrane of the vesiculæ seminales ; for they are found with analogous characters in the accessory vesiculæ of the rat, &c., which never contain animal-cules, and do not directly communicate with the vas deferens. These canals never contain similar bodies in any species. This secretion, then, is analogous to that produced by the prostatic follicles, Cowper's glands, &c. Its use is the same, and it deserves for many reasons our special attention." (Vol. ii, p. 398.)

In the former editions of this work I depended upon Lallemand for the description of these affections. Subsequent experience induces me now to believe that many of the most obstinate affections we meet with in practice depend upon previous inflammations spreading from the urethra downwards to the vesiculæ seminales, and permanently and persistently causing those interminably obstinate discharges that patients suffer from. In most of the cases complained of—when patients, on the least exertion,

[1] They have been compared to grains of sago. I am inclined to think the Professor has rather exaggerated this state of things. Modern investigation has led to a different view being taken of these bodies, and comparative anatomy teaches us that the secretion of the vesiculæ seminales is very variable in consistence : in the guinea-pig it is nearly solid, and becomes softened as soon as it comes in contact with the secretions of the vagina.

extremities in the urethra of one or both the spermatic cords may be affected. Instead of being circular, and forming little nipple-like projections, their orifices may present a stretched chink, large enough to admit a goose-quill, and there may be erosion of a sort of sphincter which surrounds them. Ulceration may attack the mucous membrane. The lining membrane may present a villous alveolar inflamed appearance, or it may become of a yellow color. Instead of being the elastic free bodies they are, they may become cartilaginous or ossified, and they may have a tortuous crooked direction." (Vol. i, pp. 11, 23.)

Fortunately for humanity, the appearances above described are rarely met with in practice. The most frequent morbid conditions of these parts depend upon inflammation attacking the vasa deferentia, consequent upon affections of the testes, and terminating in a closure, temporary or permanent, of one or both canals. In such cases the passage of the spermatic fluid is obstructed, and when the affection is permanent, sterility may be considered as beyond the control of surgery. In these cases, however, impotence, according to our definition given at page 154, does not necessarily follow. I believe that erection without subsequent emission is quite compatible with this state of occlusion of the vasa deferentia. When only one vas deferens is obstructed, of course neither sterility or impotence exists; for, as I have elsewhere stated, one perfect testis will be sufficient to carry on effectively the reproductive function, and it seldom happens that both testes become affected. Still, I believe that not unfrequently the vas deferens of one side is obstructed, and this gives rise to much local mischief, and in too many instances atrophy of the testis is the consequence, as there is no exit for the secreted semen except through the absorbent system.

TREATMENT.—The first consideration in dealing with any case of spermatorrhœa is to ascertain from which of its many causes the affection may have more especially arisen. Each patient may complain of some particular or well-marked symptom to the exclusion of all the others, though the affection itself may consist of a lesion of more than one function. It is, therefore, of great importance that this distinction should be clearly under-

19

stood. According as one or other of the functions (*e. g.* erection, emission, or the character of the emitted semen) is in fault, so must the treatment vary; what may be good in one case, may not be applicable in another. Having heard what particular symptom the patient complains of, he should be desired to make water into a glass, which should be deposited at once in a stand, to be examined at leisure. It is well at the same time to pass an olivary bougie, in order to ascertain the susceptibility of the urethra—an excellent means of arriving at an accurate diagnosis of the local state of the mucous membrane. In order to cure the affection, it is of more consequence to ascertain the *immediately* inducing local cause than the *primary cause* which may have impaired the function or originated the lesion.

Before attempting the curative treatment, the *preventive* one should be commenced. It should be ascertained if bad habits exist, and if so, the patient should be told at once that unless they are left off it is useless for the surgeon to attempt to treat him. It should, however, not be concealed from the sufferer that the means about to be employed will speedily impart such power to the will that, by his own volition, he will be capable of correcting habits which were previously beyond his control. Moderation in sexual indulgence, if not abstinence, should be enjoined on the married, and a promise to that effect obtained. It should be next ascertained whether constipation exists, whether ascarides be irritating the rectum, or if the patient suffers from varicocele. If this latter complication be present, a suspensory bandage must be worn, or, what is still better, a varicocele-ring, which the surgeon should teach the patient how to put on. The ring should be attached by a little piece of thread to the button of the drawers, otherwise it may readily slip off and be lost, and thus the testes be left without support during exercise.

The surgeon has next to determine whether the vesiculæ seminales are affected by any of the forms of irritation or inflammation spoken of in preceding pages, and if so, whether the evil may not be kept up by some of the numerous causes which, as we have seen, produce or aggravate them. The patient must do his utmost to prevent emissions taking place, and, to effect this, should have recourse to all the means spoken of at pages 231 and 236.

In the slighter cases of spermatorrhœa these remedies may alone suffice; and, as stated above, the occasional passage of an olivary bougie, or the glass tube of the instrument, hereafter to be described, will suffice to cure the patient. If, however, these plans do not succeed, and if the emissions occur, I have no hesitation in at once employing cauterization, a plan of treatment I will at once proceed to describe.

Cauterization.—In passing an instrument as above described, one or two conditions usually exists: either the instrument passes down to the vera-montanum without pain, when all at once excessive sensibility is felt in one or more spots; or the urethra is found large, patulous, and insensible, hardly seeming to feel the presence of the instrument; the former condition is, however, the one most frequently met with. Having explored the urethra, the surgeon should leave the patient quiet for that day, the only precaution taken, being that of administering a mild aperient, and desiring him to abstain altogether from stimulants or coffee. The sufferer usually prefers that the operation be performed at the surgeon's residence, and I have never found any objection to the patient returning home in a cab if the distance is not great. On the morning of the operation the patient may be allowed to eat a simple breakfast of bread, butter, or meat, but he must be strictly enjoined to abstain from fluid of any kind.

Before proceeding to perform the operation, I desire the patient to completely empty the bladder. I employ a syringe similar to the one here represented, which may be procured at Ferguson's, instrument-

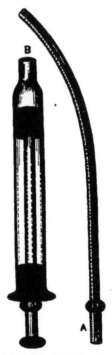

AUTHOR'S INSTRUMENT FOR CAUTERIZING THE URETHRA.

maker, Giltspur Street, Smithfield. It is made entirely of stout glass, to obviate breakage, and to avoid all decomposition of the solution of nitrate of silver. The lower part (A) can be taken off and on (at B), so as to fit into a case, thus making the instrument very portable. When put together and charged with fluid (containing a solution of ten grains of nitrate of silver to the ounce of distilled water), the instrument is passed down the urethra, the patient standing against a wall. No oil should be used, as it will interfere with the action of the caustic. The surgeon should take the precaution of folding a towel between the legs, in order to protect the trousers of the patient from being stained. The piston of the instrument is then to be forced down, at the same time that the finger and thumb of the operator's left hand compress the lips of the meatus firmly against the instrument, so as to prevent the fluid escaping from the urethra until the syringe is withdrawn, which is done as soon as the injection has been forced out of the instrument.[1] I may mention here that the syringe usually holds about two or three drachms. The pressure of the fingers on the urethra is then withdrawn, and the whole of the injected fluid passes out into the vessel which is placed to receive it. The patient may now sit or lie down in a arm chair, and remain there a quarter of an hour. The first result of the operation is to produce a warm pricking sensation at the end of the penis, which soon, however, subsides, and usually in ten minutes disappears gradually. In some cases an urgent desire to make water may come on, but as the bladder has been previously emptied, that is a fictitious want, and rapidly passes off, the patient being told to restrain the desire as much as possible. As to the pain felt after the operation, I have been over and over again assured that the suffering consequent on the application of the caustic has been much less than the patient anticipated, and in some instances it has been so slight that

[1] I should mention, that in exceptional instances I have met with some difficulty in emptying the syringe, in consequence of the strong contraction of the urethra; the fluid then, instead of passing forwards, is forced back behind the piston, and consequently does not come in contact with the mucous membrane. This, however, is of no consequence provided some of the fluid has come in contact with the morbid portion of the urethra.

the patient doubts if any caustic can have reached the affected parts.

Other patients say they have experienced none of that shock to the nervous system which interested individuals had led them to believe were sure to follow the injection of a solution of nitrate of silver, and which they had read that medical men had under-stated, in order to induce patients to submit to the operation. The first effect of the operation is to produce an oozing from the urethra, caused by the escape of a drop or two of caustic mixed with mucus, and hence a piece of linen or a folded handkerchief should be placed around the meatus to absorb the moisture, and protect the shirt from becoming stained. The patient within half an hour may be allowed to return home, but must not walk at all that day, and should swallow a copaiba capsule directly, repeating it every eight hours. Too strict injunctions cannot be given to abstain from drinking fluid of any kind until after making water, and not to pass urine until absolutely obliged. Some men can easily remain twelve hours without passing water ; a space of time which allows the caustic solution to act on the mucous membrane. When the patient is no longer able to resist the desire of making water, say twelve hours after the operation, he may drink as much weak tea, soda-water, or diluents as he pleases. Immediately after the operation he may take his usual meals, abstaining, as before said, from fluid, and confining him-self to an easy chair or sofa. During the few following hours some slight whitish discharge, like mucus, will flow from the urethra; but there will be little or no pain. When the patient first makes water there is some scalding, but the urine passes without difficulty. In some few cases, where I have reason to suppose there is an extra amount of irritability of the bladder, I have prescribed opium after the operation, but this is very rarely necessary. When the patient has made water once, he may do so as often as he likes, and each time the slight scalding will diminish, until it wholly disappears. On the day following, a tinge of blood is sometimes noticed attending the last drops of urine, but this disappears in a day or two, the urine becoming again clear. On the second or third day the copaiba capsules may be dispensed with, and the patient may commence a course of tonics with gymnastic exercises, sponging, &c., as spoken of at p. 299. Violent exercise should not be indulged in for the first few days after the operation, but a moderate walk need not be interdicted. In from four to ten days the patient may take a little claret, and subsequently resume his usual mode of life, observing, however, abstinence from tobacco or strong coffee.

Relapses.—The result of my experience proves that relapses of the local affection after cauterization do not often take place, nor is a second operation required; still every now and then cases like the following occur:—In 1853 I cauterized Mr. —— for spermatorrhœa; in August, 1854, he returned, telling me that after the last operation emissions had almost ceased, and his health improved, when within six weeks he paid attention to, and was the accepted lover of, a young lady. The marriage was to be delayed till Christmas. Lately the emissions had recurred with redoubled frequency, and he was falling into his former condition. Hearing that he would not see his intended for four months, I told him the emissions would probably cease, and if not, to take the ordinary precautions—baths, exercise (gymnastic), attention to diet and drink—and come to me a fortnight before his marriage, and I would repeat the operation.

The few cases followed by relapses are those in which men are engaged, but cannot marry from pecuniary circumstances; we meet with relapses likewise among some who will not or cannot take regular gymnastic exercise.

Beneficial effects of the operation.—The advantages of injecting a solution of nitrate of silver are so manifold, that I now never employ any other plan, and yet I have occasionally to treat some of the most obstinate forms that others have failed in curing. The operation as here described has never been attended with any unpleasant results, and I have never been called up, or been subsequently sent for, in consequence of the alarm of the patient. If the surgeon takes the precautions I have above spoken of, I have no reason to think that any untoward symptoms can arise.

I am told that in some of the books on spermatorrhœa so largely advertised in the papers, the operation is inveighed against in no measured terms. The only reply I wish to make is, that in my hands I find it most efficient and effectual, and my patients only regret that it had not been proposed to them earlier. As a result of cauterization, the patient succeeds in obtaining a control over the will which he never had before. The morbid irritability of the canal disappears, the emissions cease, and the health improves. The caustic appears to modify the local condition of the veru-montanum, and the effect is permanent *if supported by other treatment.* In this mode of operating the liquid comes in contact with every part of the canal, and does not leave untouched those depressions which escape the solid caustic, when used in Lallemand's instrument. We also have every reason to believe that by this plan the fluid enters the follicles, which are so frequently the seat of the disease, and thus tends to the cure of the complaint.

The success which has attended this mode of operating has induced me to lay aside Lallemand's instrument, which, when I commenced practice, more than thirty years ago, I used to employ. I have altered and improved the instrument I recommended on page 291 so much, that I now consider it perfect, both on the score of simplicity, usefulness, and impossibility of getting out of order.

As, however, in a work like this my readers may be desirous of comparing the one instrument with the other, I subjoin a woodcut of the catheter used by the Montpellier Professor; and I propose giving a *précis* of the mode of employing it, taken from his latest published edition.

'Lallemand's plan.—A catheter should be passed in order to empty the bladder, and to judge of the length of the urethra. This, the Professor recommends, should

LALLEMAND'S PORTE CAUSTIQUE.

be done by stretching the urethra, and, as the catheter is withdrawn, watching the moment when the water ceases to pass. Having thus discovered the length of the canal, if the finger be placed on the instrument at the point just beyond the glans penis, the exact depth to which the porte caustique should be subsequently introduced may be accurately ascertained. On the instrument which goes under Lallemand's name, there are means for measuring this distance which can be fixed by the slide seen in the woodcut.

When I was in the habit of employing Lallemand's porte caustique, I did not find it necessary to pass a catheter, as I usually enjoined a patient not to drink on the day I propose applying the instrument, and requested him to empty the bladder immediately before its introduction. It is a good precaution, moreover, to previously relieve the bowels by castor oil, or by means of an enema. The porte caustique must be prepared in the following manner:—"Fuse some broken pieces of nitrate of silver in a watch-glass held over a spirit-lamp by means of a pair of forceps, taking care to apply the heat at first at some distance, otherwise an explosion may take place; when fused, the caustic should be poured into the little cup (see woodcut), allowed to dry, and the projecting portions removed by a file; the canula must then be returned into the closed instrument, which, after being oiled, may be passed down into the bladder, the patient being in bed or lying on a sofa; a surgeon at all in the habit of passing instruments is able to distinguish when the instrument enters that viscus. The diseased part is at once known to the patient (so Lallemand states) by the instrument causing some pain. This once ascertained, the surgeon will withdraw the outer canula to the extent of half an inch, and at the same time give a rotatory motion to the inner canula containing the caustic. By this means the diseased surface is slightly cauterized, eschars are not necessarily formed, nor are any passed in the urine, and the internal canula, being drawn within the external one, cauterization is confined to the morbid structures only. Rest in the horizontal position must be enjoined, and the patient desired not to make water for some hours. If the pain comes on, a good dose of laudanum, or an enema with opium may be prescribed. For the few following days there is some pain in making water. The discharge increases, and is mixed with a little blood; but by attention to diet and rest, together with moderate doses of copaiba or cubeb capsules, these symptoms abate, and with them the emissions, although in some cases the cauterization may induce one or two escapes of semen during the following nights. Sexual intercourse must be strictly prohibited, and any cause which may originally have produced spermatorrhœa must be studiously avoided. In some cases it may be necessary to have recourse to a second or third application of the caustic; but at least ten days should elapse between each cauterization, and any accidents which may arise must be treated on general principles.

In the annexed woodcut the instrument is nearly straight, but experience taught me that such instruments cannot readily reach the bladder, and I formerly employed instruments with a considerable curve which facilitated the passage of the catheter. The cup is usually made too deep; this causes the surgeon to use not only a large proportion of caustic, but requires great care in removing the salt when it has been used. After performing the operation, I usually withdraw the canula, and soak both it and the part holding the caustic in water, or with a pointed instrument remove the nitrate of silver.

Lallemand does not assert that his plan of cauterization will be always successful. "It has succeeded," he says, "in cases where atony and debility were the prominent symptoms; less rarely when accompanied with nervous symptoms, and a strong hereditary tendency." (Vol. iii, p. 392.) Again, he says, "Two-thirds of the cases of spermatorrhœa would be beyond the resources of our art, were it not for the assistance we derive from this powerful medication." (Vol. iii, p. 406).

In twenty years, during which he was daily in the habit of using the instrument, he asserts (p. 401) that he never saw any ill consequences arise from the treatment, and I can fully bear out this statement, as far as my own experience is concerned.

Treatment after Cauterization.—As soon as the effects of cauterization have subsided, the surgeon should take steps to

scrupled to attribute the occasional loss of matches to this cause.

The diet of convalescents taking gymnastic exercise should be attended to pretty carefully. Thus, for breakfast, I prescribe cocoa and milk, and I recommend the cocoa nibs stewed down for several hours as preferable to the cocoa sold ready prepared in the shops.

Tea, coffee, and tobacco I look on as so many poisons for persons suffering under the nervous depression such as we are here speaking of. It is in vain to recommend weak tea, so I prohibit tea or coffee for breakfast, and substitute in summer seltzer-water, soda-water, or lime-water with cream or milk; those who prefer it may take claret and water, made by diluting one glass of good claret with a tumbler of water. The taking of warm fluids for breakfast is a habit that may be soon got over. I am convinced that deluging the stomach of invalids with hot strong fluid is injudicious, but at first it is somewhat difficult to induce patients to become singular and take cold fluids for breakfast. Stale bread and a moderate quantity of lean meat are advisable if the patient has a fair digestion, and if he does not feel oppressed after eating. I order luncheon for those who dine late, which may consist of a small portion of meat and stale bread, with a glass of sherry or a little bitter beer. This mid-day meal is absolutely necessary, for I find that if a man in exercise does not take nourishment in the middle of the day, he eats voraciously at dinner, and his digestion becomes impaired. I forbid late dinners, and counsel plain but wholesome diet. I·forbid fried fish, cheese, pastry, or suet-puddings, and advise only moderate quantities of meat, vegetables, and bread, with a pint of bitter beer or three moderate sized glasses of wine (claret or sherry). Both (beer and wine) should not be taken at the same meal.[1]

[1] The rules of diet that are followed in training may be interesting, though I would not recommend an invalid to attend to them strictly, except under medical advice.

One of the most successful pedestrians of the day thus described his mode of living to me. He rose early, walked one mile and a half out and back, then had a sponge-bath and took his breakfast, consisting of a cup of weak tea, or of eggs beaten up instead of milk, and a small quantity of meat.

FALSE SPERMATORRHŒA—DISEASES SIMULATING SPERMA-
TORRHŒA—QUACKS.

In the first edition of my work on "Diseases of the Urinary
and Generative Organs," I wrote a chapter entitled Syphilipho-

Then his exercise again, change of flannels, a rub down; as regards flannels
he told me he preferred wearing a tight flannel waistcoat, not merino or flannel shirts, as they felt cold if not changed. At half-past 12 he took a moderate dinner of meat, with vegetables, rice, sago, or light pudding, and a small
quantity of bottled stout. In the afternoon his exercise again; eat at five,
no meat, but a little lettuce or watercress, and at eight or nine a little arrow-
root or light supper, and then to bed in blankets. I may add that this man
was, although in very vigorous health, most moderate in sexual indulgence.

To this account I may add a description of the training that boating men
go through:

"The training of university oarsmen consists of early hours, running,
rowing, and a temperate use of the most nourishing food and drink. The
same treatment cannot be prescribed for all constitutions; but the following
seems to be about an average specimen of the way in which the month preceding the match is spent. All meet at seven a. m., and run a couple of miles
—at first, gently, afterwards at a sharp burst; this is essential, as it is the
only improver of the wind. After a tub and rub, they breakfast together in
turn at one another's rooms, and have broiled steaks and chops, bread and
butter, watercresses, and tea in moderation. A little reading fills up the
morning capitally, and keeps the mind quietly occupied; indeed, high classical attainments and good rowing often go hand in hand. At 12.30 a biscuit
and a glass of wine, and at two p. m. down to the river to row the course.
This over, they have a comfortable wash, and then dine together upon beef
or mutton sufficiently roasted, broiled, or boiled, wholesome vegetables, plain
jelly, watercresses, lettuces, and a pint of sound home-brewed ale. Pork,
veal, salted meats, made dishes, pastry, cheese, condiments, and smoking*
are forbidden. Those who are used to wine are allowed a glass or two after
dinner. All ought to be in bed shortly after ten o'clock; and, for those with
whom it agrees, the best thing to take at supper is a basin of carefully made
plain oatmeal water-gruel. But training is very ticklish work with many
men; they are apt to get feverish, and nearly the same round of food day
after day often palls. Again, about ten days after the system of training has
been begun, a period of depression sometimes occurs; this, however, is a
turning-point, and once passed, the patients feel brighter and harder. The
mentor and the coxswain strive to keep the crew cheerful and good-tempered
one with another, free from all sensations of staleness and over training. If
the cast of character includes a good low-comedy man, so much the better."
—Once a Week.

* This rule has been a little relaxed of late years, and a very moderate indulgence in tobacco has been allowed, and indeed considered beneficial.

bia in which I collected together a variety of complaints that presented many of the characteristics of true disease. Since then, a wider knowledge of these subjects has sprung up. Hypochondriacs and a large class of patients who have leisure to dwell on their morbid thoughts and feelings have, by reading the books so freely advertised in the quacks' corner of the newspapers, come to the conclusion that they are suffering under spermatorrhœa—a word with which they are now familiar. In this corner formerly five or six such advertisements directed public attention to the so-called disease; the headings of "Manly Vigor" and "Secret Diseases" have disappeared, and are replaced by the term "Spermatorrhœa,"[1] the form of sexual disease now in fashion; and as, in such hypochondriaco-misanthropic persons, the sexual feelings are generally more or less affected, the conclusion is arrived at that every one who, with a bad conscience, feels himself out of sorts, is suffering from spermatorrhœa. There is a fashion in diseases, just as there is in amusements or occupations. Patients come to us, half persuaded that they suffer in the way described, but still in doubt whether what they complain of is fancy or the real disease. In such cases we have to deal with ignorance, irritability of temper, and sometimes with true symptoms, though magnified by great exaggeration, and no inconsiderable alarm about the consequences. Conscience tells many that their previous lives have been far from faultless, and these pseudo-medical books exaggerate their indiscretion and predict the most awful consequences, describing trains of symptoms enough to frighten the most courageous. It is not difficult for my readers to surmise what must be the effect on the ignorant, the weak-minded, and those already depressed by their fears, with no friend at hand to confide in or to calm their excited feelings. Too many throw themselves into the meshes of these harpies, and the consequence is that they are fleeced to an amount that is almost inconceivable, except to those familiar with the swindling transactions of the class. As I

---

[1] Since the former editions of this book were published, its title has been pirated by more than two persons in such advertisements. On inquiry I found that it was impossible for me to prevent them from so doing.

may not have another opportunity, I would just mention a few
circumstances out of many that have come under my personal
knowledge. A student at Cambridge sought my advice suffering
from one of these sexual complaints, half real, half ideal. When
cured, he mentioned that, before coming to me he had consulted
one of the advertising firms, and after paying some £40 in fees,
was told that he could be cured only after giving his note of
hand for £300. Worn down by his alarms, fearful he should
never get well without compliance, and being of a very delicate
and susceptible disposition, he signed the agreement, and the
purport of his visit was to show me a letter in which the £300
was demanded in a very peremptory manner. I advised him at
once to put the case into a lawyer's hands; and after some hesitation on his part this was done. The interviews between the
opposing solicitors were very characteristic, but to describe them
would occupy too much space here; suffice it to say my patient's
letters were only given up after a compromise had been effected
by the payment of a sum of money.

In another case, a nobleman was asked for and gave £1000 to
one of these advertising firms; they had the impudence to ask
another £1000 some time after, under the plea that his case was
a particularly difficult one. This somewhat surprised his lordship, and the family solicitor was consulted. All attempts however, to induce the quack to refund the £1000 failed, probably
in consequence of the threats of exposure used by the firm.

The reports from the "Lancet" and the "Times" given in
the Appendix B., p. 333, will fully show the system adopted by
these pests of society.

In the more recent cases in which appropriate legal proceeding have been threatened, a moiety of the money has been
returned, without recourse to an open trial; but it too often happens that the dupe prefers losing his money to the chance of
having his weakness exposed.

This alternative, which is always threatened but never carried
into effect, however, is no longer found necessary. I once
thought that the exposure of such nefarious practices would do
good, but I now feel convinced all that can be done is to secure

a return of the money. The frequent recurrence of prosecutions for almost any disgracefully nefarious crime shows that the trial of one case does little, if anything to prevent others from occurring with exactly the same features of rascality and credulity; and I am afraid that no medical bill will cure the evil under consideration, though it may possibly change the *modus operandi.* The only efficient remedy for this system of plunder is that the profession should no longer shun the treatment of this class of diseases. It should be clearly understood by sufferers, that surgeons of repute willingly undertake the treatment of these, as well as all the other ailments to which flesh is heir, and that it is by no means necessary to resort to quacks or advertising firms. If, however, medical men desire to obtain the confidence of this class of patients, they must listen patiently to their statements, and not pooh-pooh what at first may seem fanciful.

Sufferers from false spermatorrhœa are as fully convinced that they suffer from the real ailment, the symptoms of which they complain of, as do actual invalids, and I have too much reason to think that my profession does not always appreciate these ideal sufferings. Rather with Dr. Reid in his treatise on hypochondriasis we would say: "Nothing surely can surpass the inhumanity, as well as the folly, with which patients of *this* class (sufferers from nervous diseases) are too frequently treated. We often act upon the ill-founded idea that such complaints are altogether dependent upon the power of the will; a notion which, in paradoxical extravagance, scarcely yields to the doctrine of a modern, though already obsolete writer on 'The Philosophy of Morals,' who asserted that no one need die, if with a sufficient energy he determined to live. To command or to advise a person laboring under nervous depression to be cheerful and alert, is no less idle and absurd than it would be to command or advise a person, under the direct and most intense influence of the sun's rays, to shiver with cold, or one who is 'wallowing in December's snows' to perspire from a sensation of excessive heat. The practice of laughing at or scolding a patient of this class is equally cruel and ineffectual. No one was ever laughed or scolded out of hypochondriasis. It is scarcely likely that we should elevate

rhœa complain of are frequently of the most exaggerated description; they have been mentioned in the previous pages, and it is for the medical man to decide whether they are real or assumed. Frequently they partake of both characters; there is a certain proportion of true disease which has been aggravated by fear and ill-treatment: and, I believe, as stated elsewhere (p. 69), that determination of the thoughts to a particular organ may superinduce in a greater or less degree, its functional aberration. Admitting this, great sympathy must be shown to a class of sufferers whom I fear the profession often treat with too little regard to their susceptible feelings.

In 1854 a medical student wrote to me from the country, saying that he had been twice cauterized; and he added, " supposing all further measures you may suggest for trial fail, what do you think of the operation of castration as a remedial means ?" I wrote in answer, that the operator and operated upon should be both placed in a lunatic asylum, and that I declined prescribing without seeing the patient, experience having taught me the inutility of doing so. This man represents a large class who will undergo any amount of present physical suffering to get rid of the ailment under which they believe they labor; and the probability always is, that these exaggerated accounts of disorders will turn out to be cases such as we are now speaking of—namely, real complaints enormously magnified by a highly irritable temperament. If not judiciously treated, such sufferers will assuredly end their days in asylums. I every now and then see patients who avow that they owe their lives to me, since had it not been for the assistance and sympathy held out to them, they had determined to destroy themselves—so firmly convinced had they become that they were laboring under an incurable malady, the nature of which was apparent to all beholders. It is these victories of science that make up for the disappointments medical men sometimes meet with in this sad department of the profession.

From what I occasionally witness, I am convinced that many of the suicides occurring among young men have been caused by the ineffectual treatment of supposed spermatorrhœa, and the

20

the cure. This power of imparting convictions and of controlling the will of the patient, so desired by the young surgeon, is more or less innate, but I believe can be developed by attention and extensive practice; it is frequently favored by the inferior mental acquirements of the patient, who feels comfort in reposing on one whose knowledge and truthfulness he has learned to respect.

Necessary, however, as the moral treatment I have above spoken of may be, it must often be aided by physical exertion, attention to diet, &c. In addition, local stimuli may be often necessary. When the hope can again be indulged that the dreaded impotence may, after all, be only a delusion, these and all other stimulants should be left off.

It may be advisable to interdict all sedentary and intellectual employments for the time being, and to recommend the substitution of light literature, open air exercise and change of scene; and I know of nothing that tends so much to the benefit of a patient as does a walking tour with a knapsack, particularly if he can secure the society of a pleasant companion. It is surprising what even a short trip of this kind will do, when a visit to Switzerland cannot be undertaken. It is by these means that I have been able to effect many a cure for patients whose cases had been considered hopeless.

Before closing these remarks on false spermatorrhœa, I am glad to have the opportunity of inserting a letter from the late Sir B. Brodie, sent in reply to one from a patient of this class, who has asked me to print it for the benefit of sufferers.

BROOME PARK, BETCHWORTH, SURREY.
October 14, 1854.

SIR,

Your letter reached me this morning at my country house, where I am staying for my annual vacation. I am sorry that my absence from London has caused some delay in answering it. The practice that you mention is certainly a very bad one, and if carried to excess, is often productive of very ill consequences. At the same time it must be owned, that those who have been guilty of it are often led to think that they suffer from it more than they really do by the obscene and wicked representations of quacks, whose object is to frighten young men and extort money from them. I have little doubt that you are one of the numerous class of persons who are unnecessarily alarmed. Most of the symptoms which you mention are nothing to the purpose. Many persons beside yourself have pimples on the skin, which are of no consequence, and can have nothing to do with the bad habits to which you refer, though one testicle always hangs lower down than the other. (It would be very inconvenient if it were otherwise.) You cannot have been made impotent. If you were, you could not have nocturnal emissions; to which, by the way, all young men who are not having regular sexual intercourse are more or less liable. You cannot really be very weak, as you walk seven or eight miles daily, and could, if it were necessary (as you say), walk fourteen or sixteen miles. I can perceive, however, that you are very nervous, and I dare say that you have a weak digestion. I advise you first to take the mixture of which I enclose the prescription twice daily; to live on a plain and simple diet, avoiding malt liquors, raw fruit and vegetables; and drinking merely a small quantity of sherry or weak brandy and water. Probably a visit to the sea-side will do you good. It is important that you should keep your mind well occupied. You must not expect to be relieved from nocturnal emissions until you are married.

I am, Sir,

Your obedient servant,

B. C. Brodie.

P. S. The medicine should be taken for three weeks; perhaps longer.

FOURTH PERIOD—ADVANCED LIFE.

THE FUNCTIONS AND DISORDERS OF THE REPRODUCTIVE ORGANS IN ADVANCED LIFE.

PART I.

NORMAL FUNCTIONS IN ADVANCED LIFE.

WE have seen that in childhood the generative functions should be absolutely quiescent, that even in youth the sexual powers are rather to be husbanded than taxed, and that the adult himself should be chary of exhausting those capacities which nature has given him for the extension of his species.

We have now to consider these functions, powers, and desires in advanced life; and it will appear that old age resembles youth in this, that if the elderly man wishes to preserve his intellectual faculties, health and vigor, and would enjoy a long life, he must be content with, at most, only a very moderate indulgence of the sexual passion. His motto should be, "Deposui arma miles inermis."

Fortunately for the individual, moderation is usually practised. The elderly man has generally learned from experience that the generative function cannot be wisely, or, indeed, duly exercised, before the body has attained its entire development—that it is the test of manhood, the crowning effort of maturity, and that it must diminish with a waning frame. Experience ought to have taught men that we require a sort of vital exuberance, to transmit what is superfluous to another being; and this prerogative is given to us only during the prime of our existence.

"Love," Parise,[1] that elegant writer, says, "at the decline of

[1] It has been very much the fashion to decry the French school. That many prurient ideas have been given currency to in La Belle France no one

life, should take quite a moral character, freed from all its animal propensities. In the elderly man, it is paternal, conjugal, patriotic attachment, which, without being so energetic as the love experienced in youth, still warms old hearts and old age;—and, believe me, these have their sweet privileges, as well as sometimes their bitter realities. These autumn roses are not without perfume—perhaps less intoxicating than that arising from first love, but presenting none of its dangers.

" One of the most important pieces of information which a man in years can attain is ' to learn to become old betimes,' if he wishes to attain old age. Cicero, we are told, was asked if he still indulged in the pleasures of love. ' Heaven forbid !' replied he, ' I have foresworn it as I would a savage and a furious master.'[1]

" When you see an elderly man, judicious, endowed with firm reason, whose enlightened and active mind is still capable of directing his affairs ably, and making himself useful to society,

pretends to doubt, but every reader acquainted with French literature must be aware that among its writers exist men who have given most valuable assistance in recommending moral conduct. In this category no one stands more prominently forward than M. Parise, for many years Secretary to the Royal Academy. I am proud to acknowledge the great advantage I have derived from the perusal of his work on old age. It breathes that spirit of contentment, and is written in such pure and elegant French that I fear I shall be unable, in many instances, to give the true rendering of the text; but I regret this the less if I shall induce my readers to refer to the original. I I am fully convinced they will not be disappointed, but agree with me that, among modern French literature, valuable moral instruction is to be found, draped in the most eloquent language.

[1] This saying is attributed to more than one great man of antiquity; to Sophocles, for instance. At the beginning of Plato's Republic, the merry old Cephalus says :

" I was once in company with Sophocles, the poet, when he was asked by some one, ' How do you feel, Sophocles, as to the pleasures of love? Are you still able to enjoy them ?' ' Softly, friend,' replied he, ' most gladly indeed have I escaped from these pleasures, as from some furious and savage master.' "

And again of Cato—

" Quam in eo quidam jam affecto ætate quaereret utereturne rebus venereis Dii meliora " inquit. " s. lubenter vero istinc tanquam omino agresti et furioso profugi."—Cato Maj., c. 47.

be convinced that such a man is discreet and continent, and that temperance—so justly called Sophrosyne, the Guardian of Wisdom, by the ancients—has in him a fervent admirer; in fact, he has acquired his perfect moral liberty."—*Traité de la Vieillesse*, p. 431.

M. Flourens in his "La Longévité Humaine," says—"It is at the turning point of the *physique* that the *morale* enters, in turn, upon its empire—strengthens, expands itself, and gives, as it were, a splendor to the second half of life."

"Age has a much greater effect on physiological than on sentimental love, as the latter has less need of physical force or juvenile exaltation. There are men who, always young in heart and imagination, have towards this pure love a constant devotion which, ever renewing itself, seems to reanimate instead of exhausting the vital principle."

Parise says—"It is usually at the age of fifty or sixty[1] that the generative function becomes weakened. It is at this period that *man*, elevated to the sacred character of paternity, and proud of his virile power, begins to remark that power decrease, and does so almost with a feeling of indignation. The first step towards feebleness announces to him, unmistakably, that he is no longer the man he was. He may retard the effect up to a certain point, but not entirely. This law must have its full and entire execution, '*dura lex sed lex*.' The activity of the generative organs diminishes, their functions abate, languish, and then cease entirely. The wish and the want are no longer one and the same thing; the imagination does not exercise its olden power and fascination on these organs.

"Blood now only flows in small quantities towards the testes. Their sensibility becomes blunted, and is reduced to what is sufficient for the nutrition of the parts. The scrotum is observed to become wrinkled and diminished in size, the testicles atrophy, and the complicated vascular tissues which form them become

---

[1] The Cardinal Maury is said to have told the celebrated Portal that "a man of sense past fifty ought to give up the pleasures of love, for every time he indulged in them he threw on his head a handful of earth." (Anglice, "drove a nail in his coffin.")

as for instance the deeper hollows over the eye, and by the sunken eye itself. So well are these facts known to horse-dealers, that they refuse to purchase young horses presenting these appearances, being convinced that they will not stand work, or turn out well. As far as my experience goes, no doubt can exist that old men may and do retain the power of connection under the influence of certain stimuli. Even intercourse may be, in some healthy old men, frequently repeated. Such men may have children, but experience teaches us that these infants are difficult to rear, they are not the best specimens of the English race. Too many are of a nervous irritable frame, their intellectual qualities are not equal to those of the father, and they suffer late in life from affections of the brain and nervous system. It is an undoubted fact, and is now become generally admitted, that from the moment of conception of the individual the duration of existence is, to a certain extent, pre-determined, in accordance with the organization which he has received. I think all will agree, then, that a human being born with a rich stock of force and vitality will take a greater number of years to arrive at the culmination and the term of his exist-ence, than another born under opposite conditions (even though more favorable as far as wordly externals are con-cerned). We are, therefore, forced to the conclusion that the children of old men have an inferior chance of life: and facts daily observed confirm our deductions. Look but at the pro-geny of such marriages, what is its value? As far as I have seen, it is the worst kind—spoilt childhood, feeble and preco-cious youth, extravagant manhood, early and premature death.

PART II.

DISORDERS IN ADVANCED LIFE.

FROM the above remarks we gather that the functions of the generative organs should be husbanded, not abused, in advanced life. Extreme moderation should be inculcated, and the greater the age, the greater the moderation. Entire continence—the rule of youth—is hardly less the rule of age. The transgression of this rule, indeed, in age, is more fatal than in youth. There is no superabundant stock of vitality to repair its destructive waste of error or extravagance.[1]

The greater part of mankind, however, show excessive feebleness in withstanding the abuse of the generative functions; and what surprises us most is, that those advanced in life are not always the least exposed to this reproach. It is certain that in old age, at a time when the passions have given away to reason, there are still many individuals who allow themselves to stray imprudently at the very precipitous edge of these dangerous enjoyments. They applaud themselves for postponing moderation till it is rather forced[2] than voluntary; till they stop from sheer want of vigor. What heroic wisdom! Nature, pitiless as she is, will most certainly cause them to pay dearly for the transgression of her laws; and the steady accumulation of diseases soon gives demonstrative proof of it. This result is the more certain and prompt, inasmuch as in these cases excesses are almost always of very old standing. The libertine in years has usually been dissolute in youth and manhood, so that we may trace the progress and calculate the extent of his organic deterioration.

"If we possess ever so little reflective or physiological knowledge of mankind, how can we fail to inculcate rigorously the precepts of continence, more especially as we find them calculated to maintain both the duration and happiness of our life? It is well established that, of all the powers of the economy, no one is lavished upon us by Nature with greater profusion, or, at the same time, within more clearly defined limits than this one of generation."

For the purposes of description, I shall, in the following pages, divide the functional diseases in elderly persons in the following manner, premising that it is principally from excesses that those

---

[1] See observations bearing on this question, at p. 33.

[2] Some English writer has said, "We do not forsake our vices till our vices forsake us."

that their symptoms may be slight warnings of the approach of the enemy; that, as old soldiers, they should begin to exercise a little caution.   I recall to their recollection that man has other duties which require his attention than those of reproduction.   I ask them if they have no pleasure in the luxuries of the table, or if they wish so to derange their health that their appetites shall fail.   I remind them of the saying of Bichât, "that the organ of taste is the last thread on which hangs the pleasure of living."   I repeat a few of the hints I have already detailed; and beg them to look around, and consider if their old friends who marry young wives have improved in health, or if they cannot call to mind some very notable instances of the reverse.   It occurs to them, and they do not deny, that this may be even so; and as life, and, above all, life with good health, is fully appreciated by this class of men, they become better satisfied with their position, and often appreciate my motive in thus warning them.   When I further remind them that, if nature has interdicted great sexual indulgence, it still has reserved for them many compensating pleasures; and when I hint a little later that there are other and higher enjoyments and duties which their position in society warrants and demands, we usually part pretty good friends.   I trust I have in this way been the means of rescuing many a man, who has been damaging his health in ignorance, from the dangers which beset his path, and have preserved his powers for a more prolonged discharge of his higher duties than could, under other circumstances, have been hoped for.   Lord Bacon's dictum, "Age doth profit rather in the powers of understanding than in the virtues of the affections," is not only the observation of a fact, but the inculcation of a pregnant moral.

It cannot be concealed that there are persons moving in good society (although fortunately they are few) who come to the surgeon ostensibly for other reasons, but virtually under the belief that he will prescribe something that will excite their flagging powers.   I have already alluded at length to these cases, and fully described the language which the profession does and should hold towards them.

In all such cases, the man advanced in life should be at once told that, although his powers are somewhat enfeebled, no immediate mischief has yet occurred (if the surgeon can conscientiously say so)—nature only wants rest, and all will be well. It is of great importance that the sexual fears of the elderly person should be quieted. We have seen in previous pages, the influence of the imagination on the sexual ideas. As age advances, this effect grows still stronger—it is of primary importance that the *morale* of a man should be strengthened; and I at once tell these patients most positively, that I can relieve their present sufferings; but if I attempt to renovate their sexual powers, I must exact a promise that after their convalescence they shall use them with extreme moderation. On no other terms will I undertake the case; for I tell them it is a better guarantee for their life and happiness to remain invalids as they are, than to have their organs strengthened and then to kill themselves by inches through fresh fits of excitement. I need hardly say that every upright practitioner refuses to be an accomplice in any way whatever to mere excitement. Libertinage, men should be told, is bad enough at any age; in the elderly man it is a crime, and one that no surgeon will lend himself to abet. This language held to elderly men is good in more ways than one. It proves to them that their weakened condition depends upon themselves and not upon a dreamy life alone; it "pulls them up" at a moment when they may be disposed to go astray. The assurance that their case is curable if they will only observe the ordinary rules of moderation, encourages them to leave the vicious course they may have drifted into, and regain that peace of mind the loss of which preys greatly on the bodily health of such men. No "man of the world" can pretend to be shocked by advice of this kind; many take it in good part, common sense telling them that it is reasonable, and that they must follow it if they would preserve their health.

Experience has taught me how vastly different is the situation of the class of moderate men, who, having married early, have regularly indulged their passions at longer and longer intervals as age has crept upon them, from that of widowers of some years' standing, or of men who have, through the demands of their public or other duties, been separated from their wives for prolonged periods.   The former class rarely come under the medical man's care: excesses with them are exceptional, and they are equal to the sexual shock.   On the other hand, when the latter class, after leading lives of chastity, suddenly resume sexual intercourse, they are apt to suffer greatly from generative disorders. The impression made on the nervous system, after years of rest, is calculated to impart a shock to any constitution, and this result follows with the greater certainty in those whose nervous powers are already depressed, as, for instance, by prolonged residence in the East.   These cases require great care, and their successful treatment must mainly depend on the conduct of the patient, who, by irregularities of his own,—which would appear no more than moderate in persons thoroughly sound,—may altogether frustrate every attempt to relieve him.

I was lately consulted by a gentleman of nearly seventy years of age, who, after remaining a widower many years, was captivated by the charms of a young girl.   The courtship prospered, the patient was affianced, and all appeared in satisfactory train, when he became alarmed by observing the very frequent recurrence of seminal emissions (to which he had for years been subject occasionally); and worse—which, in fact brought him to me—these emissions stained his linen with blood, a symptom which gave him great anxiety.   I pointed out to him the dangers attending this state of sexual excitement, and assured him that the treatment I should propose would avail little so long as the excitement under which he was then laboring continued, and that I dreaded the consequences.   Circumstances, however, so fell out that the marriage was broken off.   My patient soon recovered his health, and he has now occasional nocturnal emissions as before, but unattended with any hemorrhage.

The medical man may be occasionally consulted by men in years upon *the subject of marriage*, and he may be asked if his patient *may* marry.

In the former editions of this book I spoke strongly against such men marrying, and I wrote thus: "I have but one answer to all such questions.   Do it on your own responsibility ; I cannot give my sanction.   If you value life, if you consider health, if you look for happiness, I advise you to remain as you are. Much as I approve and recommend marriage to the young adult, as strongly would I forbid it to the old man."

Subsequent and more extensive experience, however, has assured me that, in the present state of civilization, there are many cases in which a man may marry late in life with great advantage. I now submit a patient who desires to marry late in life, to a close examination.   If I find him a hale person with a sound constitution, I see no objection to his settling, provided always he selects a suitable person as regards age, position, &c.   That which alone I object to, in consideration of his future health and happiness, is the uniting himself with a young, gay or volatile girl.   I am quite certain that marriage, even late in life, contributes to a man's longevity, if the woman he chooses is suitable in age, disposition, and temper.   The observations already made in this chapter particularly apply here.   If the newly-married man will but be moderate and commit no excesses of any kind, I am an advocate for his marriage, rather than that he should remain single.   The reader should recollect that in these cases the surgeon does not *advise* elderly people to marry, but he sees no valid reason why an attachment already formed should be broken off because the bridegroom is advanced in life.   I am cognizant of many instances of persons who are now living very comfortably and happily who have married late in life.   In these instances no ill consequences have happened.   If, however, an elderly man is disposed to marry beneath him, or to contract marriage with a young and worldly woman, I think his medical adviser should do all in his power to dissuade him and to warn him of the danger he is about to incur.   Nevertheless, experience teaches us that the advice is but little heeded.   I am well aware that many cases can be cited in which men have married late in life, and had families.   Undoubted instances of virility at the age of nearly one hundred years are on record ; but in these cases the general bodily vigor has been preserved in a very remarkable degree. The ordinary rule seems to be, that sexual power is not retained by the male to any considerable amount after the age of sixty or sixty-five.

The impunity with which some elderly men continue the practice of sexual intercourse is certainly surprising; still abuse or excess, whichever we may term it, must sooner or later tell its tale. In some, its effects assume the form of hypochondriasis, followed by all the protean miseries of indigestion; in others, of fatuity; in the more advanced stages, paralysis or paraplegia come on, accompanied by softening of the brain, and its attendant consequences. What in early life was followed by temporary languor, is in age not unusually followed by the train of symptoms alluded to above; and when we are called in, it is too late to do aught but palliate them.

I am becoming every day more convinced that many of the affections of the brain, under which elderly persons suffer, and from which a certain proportion annually perish, are caused by excesses committed at a time when the enfeebled powers are unequal to supporting them, and I think it the duty of the medical profession to put such sufferers in possession of these facts. Kind advice and sympathy would thus, I am sure, save the valuable life of many a man who errs from ignorance. Let us listen to the warning voice of one who, as I have before said, has written the best work on diseases of old age. Parise is inveighing against ill-assorted marriages of elderly persons. " There are great risks run; for in the extreme disparity of age, and oftentimes of condition—as when the man is rich and the girl is young—Nature avenges herself by spreading scandals, doubts about paternity, and domestic troubles; everything is at variance, age, disposition, character, tastes and amusements. ' What shall I do with him, and what will he do with me?' said a clever young girl of eighteen, whose parents wished her to marry an old gentleman. With regard to health and vital force, it is easy to foresee what will become of them in these unequal marriages, where a young and fresh girl is ' flesh of the flesh' of a man used up from age, and mayhap from excesses. Evidently she commits a suicidal act more or less certain or rapid. On the other hand, experience shows that the elderly man who thus risks his repose

21

and his existence, speedily finds his health grievously affected; and with what justice may not the lines of the poet Hardy be applied to his case—

        ' " ' On ne se servira que d'um même flambeau,
           Pour te conduire au lit, et du lit au tombeau.' "

"Would you," continued Parise, "know the difference between love in youth and in old men ? It is this, 'of a truth *great folly appertaineth to the first love, but great feebleness to the last.*' Hereby hangs a tale, for sudden danger lies in the path, and the siren sings upon the very verge. Blessed should the old man deem himself who can put up with calmness, happiness, and reason, instead of craving after those senile accessions of delirium too often the parents of regret and remorse without end. The chastisement of those who love the sex too much is to love too long. Is Nature silent ? 'Tis that she would not speak ? Would you provoke or excite her ? It is a crime against her—a crime for which she will some day claim a deep revenge. Why, then, not listen to the voice of wisdom—for those who sit at her feet, and listen to her awful counsels, shall be delivered from strong passion, and many sore straits and much folly ?"

Let the elderly man, then, pause and reflect, that a human sacrifice, either male or female, is generally bound to the horns of the altar that sanctifies such marriages. In the present state of society, with our manners, passions, miseries, *man does not always die—he sometimes destroys himself.* And the sort of union I have touched upon is one of the most ingenious devices of men to expedite that natural friction by which our vital forces are expended in the course of threescore years and ten.

It was thus I wrote in composing the last edition of this book, and I cannot even now characterize in stronger terms the danger an old man incurs in contracting unequal marriages ; but I would here repeat what I said at page 320.

I see no objection to an elderly man marrying a woman in a rank compatible with his own, and whose age is in proportion to the average we have laid down at page 127.

In these cases, excesses are not likely to occur, and I feel convinced that an old bachelor by remaining an old *roué* may run greater risk than by marrying. In either case I should say avoid excess; but I no longer set my face against marrying late, only against the excesses to which it may lead. Not a few such marriages about which I have been consulted have turned out well, and have led to much mutual domestic happiness.

CHAPTER II.

FUNCTIONAL DISORDERS IN PERSONS WHO KNOW THE CONSE-
QUENCES OF SEXUAL EXCESSES, BUT CANNOT CONTROL THEIR
PASSIONS.

This is a class of persons the consulting surgeon occasionally meets with who are deserving of great sympathy. Their passions depend too frequently on a state of excitement over which they themselves have no control, although its origin may be traced to their own excesses. These patients come to ask our assistance, not with any object of obtaining power, but because they suffer from urgent desire, which a careful examination of the case often convinces us is fictitious, and dependent upon some irritation going on in one part or other of the canal. In some persons, a full bladder will occasion it; in others, irritation about the rectum, proceeding from worms or hæmorrhoids; in others, again, acidity of the urine will induce a morbid craving that is often most distressing to the sufferer. Often the affection depends upon neuralgia of the bladder, or stone in that viscus. In other instances, I have seen reason to attribute it to some affection of the skin covering the generative organs, causing local excitement. It is all very well to desire such patients to resist these morbid desires, but until appropriate local treatment is prescribed, there can be little hope of amendment. Some few think that this unnatural excitement is healthy. They pride themselves upon it, appear astonished at the surgeon wishing to remove the cause, and cannot comprehend that their constitutions have been much reduced by the fatigue which the organs have undergone. Ultimately for the most part, common sense triumphs, and they feel intensely grateful for the relief they obtain.

The surgeon must acknowledge, however, that these affections are frequently very rebellious. The duration of disease, prolonged residence in warm or unhealthy climates, or the fact of the sexual passions having been allowed unrestrained liberty, have often brought the constitution of the elderly man into a very irritable state; still, great amelioration may be surely promised. The means of cure cannot here be dwelt upon. They must depend not only on the particular affection present, but the case must be treated on the ordinary principles of surgery.

CHAPTER III.

FUNCTIONAL DISORDERS IN DEBAUCHEES WHO, HOPING TO SUPPLY THE LOSS OF POWER CONSEQUENT ON THEIR PREVIOUS EXCESSES, PREFER TO STIMULATE THE REPRODUCTIVE ORGANS FOR THE PURPOSE OF GRATIFYING THEIR ANIMAL PASSIONS.

Again, we quote Parise: "Unfortunately there are those who, either more infatuated, more helplessly drifting on the tide of passion, or more depraved, use all their endeavors to realize desires which it is no longer possible to satisfy, unless by a forced compliance of the organs. Not only has the energy—the superfluous vitality of early days—disappeared, but the organic power of reproduction is nearly obliterated. Is all over then? *Credat Judærus non ego.* It is now that Venus Impudica lavishes on her *used-up* votaries her appetizing stimulants to vice and debauchery. The imagination polluted with impurities, seeks pleasure which reason and good sense repudiate. There are instances of debauched and shameless old age which, deficient in vital resources, strives to supply their place by fictitious excitement; a kind of brutish lasciviousness, that is ever the more cruelly punished by nature, from the fact that the immediately-ensuing debility is in direct proportion to the forced stimulation which has preceded it.

"Reduced to the pleasures of recollection, at once passionate and impotent, their sensuality may kill, but cannot satiate. There are such old libertines who are constantly seeking after the means of revivifying their withered, used-up organism, as if that were possible without imminent danger. The law of nature is without appeal. To submit to it is the result of great good judgment, and the reward is speedy. But submission is no invariable rule, and persons of prudence and chastity have but faint conception of the devices to evade it, of the folly, caprice, luxury, immodesty, the monstrous lewdness and indiscribable saturnalia of the senses which are the result. The surgeon alone knows from the confession of his patients, or surmises from his experience, to what a depth corruption will descend, and the evils which will follow, particularly in large capitals. One of the most common means of excitement employed by these senile Lovelaces is change—variety in the persons they pursue. What is more fatal to the *organism?* Extreme youth is sacrificed to these shameless old men. The full-blown charms of fine women no longer suffice—they address themselves to mere children, to the great scandal of our manners, and of all that these victims of debauchery hold dear and sacred. Nevertheless, let it be remarked, it is seldom—very seldom—that punishment comes *pede claudo;* old age, which disease changes every day into decrepitude—often sudden death, and death that lasts for years, a consequence of cruel infirmities—prove the justice of Nature." (Parise, p. 423.)

It would be well if the above picture, sketched, of course, from Parisian society by a distinguished French physician, were inconsistent with experiences gathered elsewhere.

Regret it as we may, medical men of large experience must acknowledge that human nature presents much the same features under all climates, and in London as elsewhere. Virtue and sin, refinement and vice, appear to me to herd together and to grow intense, *pari passu* with civilization.

When a young man, without any redeeming qualities, has run through a career of debauchery, when his adult age is but a new lease of similar associations, the necessity for additional excite-

for a lunatic asylum, as in all other respects their conduct appears to be sane. Observing, as these persons do, all the other usual *convenances* of society, there is yet a something about them which marks them as thralls of a debasing pursuit. It is an error, however, to suppose that they often suffer from venereal disease. Your old *débauchés* know too well the parties they have to deal with, and every precaution is taken to avoid the consequences. They are living and suffering spectres whom, as some clever writer has observed, "Death seems to forget to strike, because he believes them already in the tomb."

I very much question if, with their disordered brains, the fear of punishment will deter such men from crime. These satyrs are reduced to so morbid a condition, that the very chance of exposure seems to add a last stimulus to their debased inclinations. No other reason can, it seems, be given to explain why these rich old *débauchés* should choose places of public resort for their vile practices, when all that is there performed could by the aid of money and existing agencies, be done in secret. It would seem as though stolen sweets and covert joys had lost their charm; and the chance of evading the law had become the fascinating novelty. Hence the risk, the subsequent detection, and the public discovery of the practices of those whose *penchants* have long been known to the police. It is a form of aberration of intellect to which libertinage is subject; and seems to show into what a morass of defilement unrestrained sexual excitement may finally lead its victim.

It may, perhaps, be thought singular in my suggesting a moral based upon such vile practices as the above, but allusion to them may not be without benefit to those beginning life; and I would say, let those persons take warning who with an active imagination once enter upon a career of vice, and dream that at a certain spot they can arrest their progress. It is an old tale, and often told, that, although the slope of criminality be easy and gradual, it is still "le premier pas qui coute;"—and he who launches himself on such a course, will acquire, as he goes, velocity and force, *until at last he cannot be stayed.*

not likely to do so.   Once in the vicious circle, he *must*, sooner
or later, find a confidant in our profession; it is then that the
judicious surgeon may step in, and by firm but feeling language
he often can, and, if he can, I need not say he ought to try and
put a stop to this career of iniquity.   There are moments of regret, there are periods of suffering, when a word of advice can
be given ; and if the true consequences of unrestrained licentious-
ness be urged, the easy descent from the comparative happiness
and respectability may be arrested, and the ignominious end
averted.   I admit the difficulty.   I am well aware that such interference may be thought impertinent ; but no man can so well
interfere or has such opportunities of expostulation as the medical
man.   If he do not, few else can, and no one else will.   His duty
to his country as a citizen, to his patient as a friend, calls upon
him loudly, I think, to act the part of a kind and sympathetic
adviser,

With his store of argument based upon experience, and his
ample choice of opportunities, it is hard to say how often the
well-intentioned professional man may not be the means of saving
a fellow-creature from the prison, the poor-house, or the lunatic
asylum ; and of rescuing from base perversion the noble faculties
lent by the Almighty for the fulfilment of His first command to
Man.

APPENDIX.

A.

Suprà, p. 186.

PRESCRIPTIONS.

I HAVE thought it better for many reasons, to collect a few of the more usual prescriptions in an Appendix, than to encumber the text with them.

℞. Ferri Citratis c. Strychniâ, gr. iij ;
Quinæ Disulph., gr. j.
M. fiat pilula ter die sumend.

℞. Ferri et Quinæ Citratis, ℈ij ;
Liq. Strychniæ, B. P., ℳxlv ;
Syrupi, ʒvj ;
Aquæ ad ℥iv.
M. fiat mist. cujus cap. coch. ampl. ex cyath. vin. aquæ ter die.

℞. Ferri Ammon. Citratis, ʒi ;
Ammon. Sesquicarb., ʒj ;
Ætheris Chlorici, ʒij ;
Sp. Lavandulæ c., ʒvj ;
Aquæ Piment. ad ℥vj.
M. sumat coch. j amplum ex cyath. vin. aquæ horâ 11 a.m. et horâ 4ta p. m. quotidie.

℞. Acid. Phosph. dilut.,
Syrup. Zingiberis,
Syrup. Aurant, āā ℥ss.
M. fiat mist. cap. coch. j. min. ter die ex cyath. vin. aqua.

℞. Syrup. Ferri Phosph., ʒj ;
Acid. Phosph. dilut., ʒiss ;
Mist. Acaciæ, ℥iij ;
Sp. Aurant, ℥ss ;
Aquæ Anethi ad ℥viij. M.
Two table-spoonfuls to be taken twice a day, at eleven and four, with a table-spoonful of Cod-Liver Oil.

℞. Sqdæ Hypophosph., ʒvj ;
　Syrup. Aurant., ℥ij :
　Aquæ ad ℥vj. M. Capiat cochl. med. j ter die.

℞. Ext. Cannabis Indicæ, gr. j ;
　Pulv. Glycyrrhizæ, q. suf.
M. ft. pil. horâ somni sumend.

℞. Ol. Phosphorat., ℥j ;[1]
　Ol. Morrhuæ, ℥vij. M.
A teaspoonful, gradually increased, for a dose.

℞. Tinct. Cantharidis, ʒiss ;
　Sp. Lavandulæ co., ℥j ;
　Ætheris Chlorici, ʒj ;
　Aquæ ad ℥viij. M. ft. mist.
Two table-spoonfuls to be taken three times a day ; at
　eleven, four, and at bed-time.

℞. Chloralis Hydratis, ʒj ;
　Syrupi Aurantii, ℥j ;
　Tinct. Aurantii, ʒiv ;
　Aquæ ad ℥iij. M.
A dessert-spoonful for a dose.

In case where a local stimulant is necessary, I have found the
following answer well :

℞. Linim. Sinapis comp., ℥ss ;
　Eau de Cologne, ℥j. M. ft. embrocatio.

---

[1] ℞. Phosph., gr. vj ;
　Ol. Amygdalæ, ℥j. M.
　　　　　Pruss. Ph.

B.

Suprà, p. 302.

EXPOSURE OF THE QUACK SYSTEM.

BLOOMSBURY COUNTY COURT.

July 30*th*, 1857.

(Before Mr. LEFROY, DEPUTY-JUDGE.)

—— *v.* KAHN.

This was an action brought by the plaintiff, a clerk in a mercantile house, against the defendant, Dr. Kahn, proprietor of the Anatomical Museum in Coventry Street, to recover the sum of 20*l.*, alleged to have been fraudulently obtained under the following singular and extraordinary circumstances.

The case has excited a great degree of interest in the medical world, and the court was crowded with spectators, anxious to hear the result of the trial. Amongst the company were several eminent medical practitioners.

Mr. BOWEN MAY, solicitor of Russell Square, appeared for the plaintiff; and Mr. BERNARD, counsel, conducted the defence.

In opening the case, Mr. MAY said,—This action is brought to recover the trifling sum of 20*l.* The particulars of the plaintiff's demand set out that it is for damages occasioned by the defendant's improper treatment during the months of August and September, 1856, whilst employed by the plaintiff to cure him of a complaint under which he was then laboring, whereby the plaintiff was put to useless expense and pain, and the plaintiff claims the said sum of 20*l.* for money had and received, and fraudulently obtained of the plaintiff by the defendant.

The learned counsel for the defence here suggested the propriety of all females leaving the court, which having been complied with,

Mr. MAY proceeded.—The action is to recover the sum of 20*l.*, fraudulently obtained from the plaintiff, but in spirit it is brought for the good of the public and society at large. The plaintiff is clerk to an eminent firm in the city, and is a very respectable man. The defendant is one of those gentlemen who live upon human nature, by frightening weak-minded people, and reducing them to such a state of alarm as to be enabled to act upon their credulity. He is not a qualified practitioner, but avows to the world that he is a physician, and it is under that representation I shall show that the public are induced to go to him. Directly he obtains his fee, he does not care one farthing for the cure of the patient, and he also presupposes that persons are laboring under "spermatorrhœa." Now, your Honor, this young man in a weak moment went to Dr. Kahn, and the first thing Dr. Kahn said to him was. — You have spermatorrhœa : what money have you? You see this is a very dangerous disease, and I am the only one who can cure it ; but if I cure you. it must be for a good amount. However. as you are a poor man. I'll do it for 20l." And nothing more was said then. but a panacea was given—supposed to contain antimony. the effect of which is to depress the patient to such an extent. that a person laboring under its influence for any period would believe anything. Then by a microscope the doctor discovered some animalculæ. This is one of the microscopic dodges. which frighten nervous people. He produces this before the man. who said, "What am I to do?" He answered. — I shall want 50l." Then when he finds this poor young man is acted on in this way, who could not give 50l., as he said, the doctor exclaimed, " Your brains are passing out into your water. and you will die." (Laughter.) And thus the young man was reduced to that state of melancholy that he would believe anything that was told him, and when he came again. he found that he was worse instead of better. No man goes to these quacks unless his mind has been acted upon previously, and then nothing is too gross for him to be made to believe. Now, it is a singular fact, that directly the plaintiff left off the medicine. he got better. He went to a regular practitioner, and in about three weeks he was well. Sir, I will show to you that this is a common occurrence with Dr. Kahn. I shall show you a case where he got a heavy sum of money from a person under precisely similar circumstances

THE DEPUTY-JUDGE.—No, no ; that will be quite unnecessary, because we are trying this case upon its merits.

Mr. MAY.—But, your Honor, I shall show complicity, not only that this case is a fraud, but that it comes forth with a fraudulent intent. I shall satisfy you that this defendant lives upon the vitals of young men by the money that he obtains in this identical way. I shall examine Mr. Hancock, a gentleman of great repute as a surgeon to the Charing Cross Hospital—

THE DEPUTY-JUDGE.—Your case is, that he really obtained money by fraudulent pretences.

Mr. MAY.—If I bring an action against an unqualified man, I must show that he professes that for which he is not legally qualified.

THE DEPUTY-JUDGE.—But you have no right to go into other cases where he obtained money ; that has nothing to do with the present case ; and if you prove what you have opened, I do not see that it is necessary to prove anything more. You surely have opened quite enough.

Mr. MAY.—This is a matter of public importance. It is not merely a question of 20l., which only forms a little ingredient. The sum obtained was 51l. ; the first sum was 1l., and he gradually gets money until he obtains that amount in the aggregate, which is the customary practice of these charlatans. If he were a qualified man, then he would not be entitled to what he has charged. I shall show that the most he can charge is a guinea ; whereas we pay 50l. for not being cured, but on the contrary, actually being made infinitely worse. The fact is, he is one of these advertising quacks, and it is not for the trifling sum that we come here to-day; but we wish, by the judgment of your Honor, which I have no doubt will be in favor of the plaintiff, to suppress this monstrous system of traffic and trading upon young men. I shall prove to the Court that he is in the habit of getting thousands of pounds from clergymen and other young men who are ashamed to state what their cases of disease are. I shall also prove that the plaintiff had scarcely any malady upon him at all; but that he was reduced to this state merely for Dr. Kahn's purpose, that of putting money into his pocket. First, I shall call the plaintiff, to show your Honor that he was to be cured for 20*l.*; that there was a compact; and medical evidence to prove that the patient's symptoms could only be produced by the medicines administered to him by the defendant; and I shall satisfy you that when persons labor under disease produced by such treatment, they fall into a state which occasionally leads to insanity. Perhaps the most atrocious part of this case is, when the young man said, "You've not cured me; give me back my money!" and the doctor replied, "If you dare ask for that, I shall accuse you of masturbation" (sensation), which was utterly false, and a piece of rascally conduct on the part of the defendant.

The DEPUTY-JUDGE.—Oh! even if it were true, it would be a monstrous thing for a medical man to assert. (A burst of applause for a moment followed this remark from the Bench, but was immediately repressed.) I say, whether it be true or not, it is a breach of confidence, and a monstrous assertion to make.

The plaintiff was then sworn and examined by Mr. May.

I believe you went to consult Dr. Kahn?—I went in the month of August, 1856.

Did you believe he was a regular practioner?

Mr. BARNARD.—I object to that question.

Mr. MAY —In what capacity did you go to him?—I went to consult him about my health.

But for that you would not nave gone to him?—No; and I waited an hour before I could see him. He asked me what was the matter; and I told him that I had had the "clap," and that I did not think that I was cured of it.

Was there anything important the matter with you at that time?—Nothing at all, except when I went to the water-closet there was a little secretion came from me, and I told him that, and he said,—"Let me look at it"—"Let me look at you." So I let my trousers down, and he put his hand there, and said, "You have been committing self-abuse; you have got spermatorrhœa." And I said, "I have not."

Now, I ask you if you ever did so?—I never did it in my life; and the doctor then said, "My fee is a guinea;" and he said, "my charge to cure you of spermatorrhœa is 20*l.*," after having received the guinea. I called again, and he gave me a little case with six small bottles in it. I had not spermatorrhœa at that time. I took him 10*l.*, and afterwards 9*l.* Altogether I gave him 21*l.* 1*s.*; and he said, "I have got your medicine prepared for you. You go home now, get into a room, and never stir out for eight-and-twenty weeks; and take

I heard about two months afterwards that it was not Dr. Kahn, but his brother. Kahn did also attend me, though.

Were you a married man at this time?—No, a widower, and had a child.

What have you been doing since?—Well, I do as a good many men do; I run astray sometimes. It was the first time. All I told Dr. Kahn was, that when I went to the water-closet there was some secretion come from me, and that I had the clap. I felt it in June, and I should think it was on for more than six weeks.

How came you to go to Dr. Kahn?—A friend of mine had gone to one o his lectures, and he brought one of his books with him.

Now, what are you?—I am a clerk.

In whose employ?

Mr. MAY.—Don't tell him.

The DEPUTY-JUDGE.—Surely that is unnecessary. It is a needless exposure.

I object to say; but I will write it down. However, if I must say, I will do so openly in court. I am employed by the ——, the railway contractors in the ——, and I have been there eleven years.

You married again?—Yes.

When did you marry? Last week.

Had you consulted any other man at all before you went to Dr. Kahn?—No, I had not.

By the COURT.—Altogether I saw him about eighteen times, and I paid three times the amount.

Re-examined by Mr. MAY.—Where did you see this second man who called himself Dr. Kahn? Was it at defendant's house, at 17, Harley Street?—Yes.

And when you saw the real "Simon Pure" had you any conversation with him?—No.

The DEPUTY-JUDGE.—When you saw the real Dr. Kahn was any thing said about his brother's treatment?—He said his brother was ill, and he would prescribe for him.

Did you know Dr. Kahn was a lecturer?—No.

Dr. M'CANN sworn, and examined by Mr. MAY.—I have heard the history of this plaintiff, and in my opinion the depression, lassitude, and state of the patient would be produced by—

Mr. BARNARD (counsel)—I object to the question and answer being given in this way.

Mr. MAY.—What effect has antimony, Dr. M'Cann, upon a patient under such circumstances?

Question objected to.

Would the proper medicine for spermatorrhœa produce the effect that was produced upon the plaintiff?

The DEPUTY-JUDGE.—What is the proper medicine?—That would depend upon the causes from which it arose, but tonics and chalybeates generally ought to be given.

22

The Deputy-Judge.—The important part of this case is the threat to disclose it. It does not signify whether the man had it or not. The defendant would have no right to extort money under that threat to him. (A letter was here read to show that the plaintiff had admitted having practised masturbation from the time he was eighteen up to the present period of his life. The document was from the defendant's solicitor: and the plaintiff being again called, declared that he never said he attributed the symptoms of his case to self-abuse.)

Examination of Mr. Acton resumed.—Can you tell from the examination of a patient whether he is guilty of that practice?—It is impossible.

The Deputy-Judge.—Would the practice produce spermatorrhœa?—It is one of the many causes.

What is the effect of giving small doses of antimony to the patient?—It has a very depressing effect, such as described by the plaintiff.

Was there any semen passing from the patient while he was under your treatment?—None, sir.

Are yellow soap and alum the proper treatment?—It is a very homely remedy, but it is not a medical one. I should think it would be highly irritating.

From the known properties of those two articles, would they be likely to irritate?—Yellow soap is an irritant, and alum is the same.

The Deputy-Judge.—That is important.

Cross-examined by Counsel.—Had the pimples disappeared?—Yes, because twelve months had elapsed. I should be sorry to put either alum or yellow soap to any irritable sore.

Mr. May proposed to show that the name of Dr. Kahn was not in the "London Medical Directory" of licensed practitioners, when an objection was taken by counsel in which the Court concurred.

Dr. Semple was sworn and examined by Mr. May.—I am a physician and also a surgeon, and until lately was one of the examiners at the Apothecaries' Hall. All licensed medical men have their names recorded in the "London and Provincial Medical Directory."

Mr. Barnard.—I object to the statement.

The Deputy-Judge.—It would be hard to say that a man was not a barrister because his name was not in the "Law List." I don't see that the matter is worth much.

The Witness.—I entirely agree with the two preceding witnesses as to alum and soap being irritants. The soap contains a strong alkali.

The Deputy-Judge.—Supposing a man were suffering from spermatorrhœa, what do you say to ordering him to remain in a room for twenty-eight weeks? —Most decidedly improper in my opinion.

Mr. May.—It would tend to promote the very disease under which he was said to be laboring?—Quite so.

Would pork be objectionable?—Not at all.

You have heard the description from the patient. How long with the constitution of a horse, ought the complaint to have been before it was cured?

such things are allowed.　The case in question is simply an illustration of a system so ruinous, so devastating, so fatal to its victims, that it calls loudly for legislative interference.　Laws, however framed, will probably be inadequate to altogether suppress these outrages upon humanity; but legislation may do something to mitigate and arrest them.　If we are to have laws for the protection of women, and for the suppression of obscene publications, why should we not have an Act of Parliament to suppress a traffic which, in its consequences, is equally detrimental to the health and happiness of a large portion of the public?"

SINCE the aboved recited case was published a still more striking disclosure of the quack system has been brought before the public, and I think I shall not do amiss if I extract it in full from the columns of the "Times" of Friday, November 25th, 1864.

CENTRAL CRIMINAL COURT.

November 24th.

OLD COURT.

(Before Mr. Baron BRAMWELL.)

John Osterfield Ray, or Wray, and William Anderson, respectably dressed men, were arraigned on an indictment charging them with having feloniously sent a letter to Montague Augustus Clarke, demanding 150*l.* from him, with menaces.

Mr. Metcalfe and Mr. Hume Williams were counsel for the prosecution; Mr. Sergeant Ballantine, Mr. Ribton, and Mr. F. H. Lewis defended the prisoner Ray, and Mr. Kemp defended Anderson.

The prosecutor and the principal witness was Montague Augustus Clarke. He said, in answer to Mr. METCALFE,—I am a captain in the 50th Regiment, the depôt of which is quartered at Parkhurst, the regiment itself being now on service in New Zealand.　In consequence of seeing some advertisements I came from Parkhurst to London, to consult Dr. Henery, in Dorset Street.　I went there, and saw the prisoner Ray, who said he was Dr. Henery.　This was about the 17th of August last year.　I consulted him about a disease from which I was suffering, and he gave me a little advice.　It was very little indeed.　He said he would forward me some medicine.　I asked what his charge was, and he replied "1*l.* 1*s.* for advice, and 10*l.* 10*s.* for the medicine."

wrote a letter to Dr. Henery, stating that a gentleman, describing himself as his agent, had made a claim on me for 150*l.*; that I was quite unaware of owing him such a sum, and that I should be obliged by his sending me the particulars, in order that I might send them to my legal adviser, addressing me to the care of Messrs. Cox. I received a letter from him in answer. [It was read as follows]:

"MEDICAL INSTITUTION, 53 DORSET STREET, PORTMAN SQUARE,
"LONDON ; *Sept.* 26*th.*

SIR,—I regret exceedingly to have to inform you that your letter did not reach me until Saturday night ; otherwise it would have received my immediate attention. Nevertheless, I have to remind you that you promised the gentleman who waited upon you at Parkhurst that you would call at Dorset Street; therefore I do not understand your giving us so much trouble in the matter. I have to inform you that my claim for 150*l.* is for medical advice and medicine for spermatorrhœa brought on by self-pollution. If you will satisfy my claim without further trouble I will give you a receipt in full of all demands, or sign any paper that you may please to draw up, so that you shall not be troubled again by

"Your obedient servant,
"A. F. HENERY.

"P. S.—I called at Cox and Co.'s this morning, and found that you were there on Saturday, so therefore I hope this will reach you there." •

I also handed that to my legal adviser. On the 5th of October I received another letter signed "H. Wilson," and which, I think, is the handwriting of the prisoner Anderson :

"WARBURTON'S HOTEL, NEWPORT ; *Oct.* 5*th,* 1864.
"Private Sitting Room, No. 4.

"SIR,—I am here expressly from London to see you with a view to effect a settlement, if possible, of Dr. Henery's claim ; and anticipating your refusal to see me at your quarters is the reason I have penned this and I would recommend you to do so at once, for, rely upon it, I don't intend journeying here again for nothing. Your letter from your solicitor has been received, and I have that and some from yourself with me. Now, supposing I were to inform you application will be made at the War Office, with explanation of your case ; and if we were to do so you know what the consequence would be ; or supposing I were to inform you that I expect to be in your neighborhood in Scotland next week, and that I don't intend leaving here in the event of your still persisting in your refusal to pay without making it known in the neighborhood for what purpose I am here. I am in no hurry, and will allow you time to reflect whether it will be better to pay Dr. Henery's legal and just claim or submit to exposure of your filthy case. I would inform you I have waited upon one of the head solicitors in Plymouth since I saw you, in reference to a claim we had upon his son, and on our explaining what we would do in the event of his not paying us, he soon saw the force of what we said and paid us at once. Now, the reason I did not tell you what we intended

23

doing in the event of your not paying when I was here before was because you promised to call in Dorset Street, and relying on your word as a gentleman was the only reason I did not do so.

"Yours obediently,

"H. WILSON.

"P. S.—It is useless for you to pretend you are not in quarters, for I know you to be there (and was there last night when I called) before I left London."

In that letter there is an allusion to Scotland. My father resides there and some other of my friends. I had written from Scotland to Dr. Henery once while I was receiving medicine from him, so that he knew my address there. I placed that letter in the hands of my legal adviser.

By Mr. RIBTON, in cross-examination.—When I consulted him I was suffering from a malady, and I described my symptoms to him. The interview lasted about five minutes. The box he first sent me contained twelve bottles of medicine. I did not take it all. He gave me certain directions as to regimen, exercise, bathing, and the like, but only such as I had followed all my life. I acknowledged to Anderson owing Dr. Henery 10l. 10s. for a box of medicine, which I was prepared to pay, but I would not pay him any more. I believed I was suffering then from the disease called spermatorrhœa.

Re-examined by Mr. METCALFE.—I was in the Crimea, and was badly wounded in the head. I should think my constitution was injured there.

ALEXANDER THOMPSON, Clerk in the London and Westminster Bank, deposed that the prisoner Wray kept an account at the bank, and that the endorsement on the checks of Captain Clarke was in the handwriting of Wray.

Sergeant WHITE, of the N. division, deposed that on the 22d of October the case against the defendant Anderson was heard at Marlborough Street Policecourt. Anderson appeared, but Henery did not. A warrant was issued for his apprehension, and witness went to his house in Dorset Street, Portman Square, and found him in bed. He said he was too ill to get up. Witness replied, "Nonsense; I saw you out yesterday, and you must go." He answered, "My name is not Henery; if the summons had been made out in the name of Wray I should have appeared." Witness pulled off the bedclothes, and found him partly dressed.

This was the case for the prosecution.

Mr. Baron BRAMWELL held that there was no evidence to sustain the first count for publishing a malicious libel, while the second fell to the ground on account of the venue, the alleged offence having been committed in the county of Hampshire.

The jury then, under the direction of the learned Judge, returned a verdict of *Not Guilty*.

The prisoners were then arraigned on a charge of conspiracy by divers false pretences and subtle means and devices to obtain large sums of money from the prosecutor, and also of threatening to publish a libel concerning him with a view to extort money.

Mr. RIBTON, addressing the jury on behalf of the prisoner Wray, submitted that there was not a tittle of evidence to show that Wray was responsible for anything that had been done by Anderson in the country. He admitted that the letter written by Anderson from Warburton's Hotel was a threatening letter, and that its purpose was to get money from Captain Clarke by menace, but he utterly denied that there was any evidence that Wray was cognizant of that letter being about to be written, or that he ever gave any instructions to Anderson to write it. They could not, either in principle or in law, hold the principal responsible for all the acts of his agents, but only for those acts which he had directed to be done. No doubt Captain Clarke at that time was laboring under some disease. If he were not, then indeed, there would be a false pretence, but we could not understand how a false pretence could be alleged when the origin of the demand was admitted by the prosecutor himself to be true. It is well known that certain members of the medical profession devoted themselves to a particular description of disease, and that they advertised in the papers, and he was not aware that there was any disgrace in their doing so. Captain Clarke, seeing Wray's or Henery's advertisement, went to him and received medicine and advice. It was idle, therefore, to say that there was any false pretence. It had not been shown what were the ingredients of which the medicine was composed. In all probability it was a strong tonic, and intended to do Captain Clark good, and charging for it more than he ought was not an offence on the part of Wray. Nay, it had been mentioned that within the last three years a member of his own profession had refused to come into that court unless they gave him 1000 guineas (a laugh), and he understood that the gentleman who did come on that occasion received a very large sum. Then in what way could Wray be affected by the letters which had been read? The letter of September 26th, 1864, had formed the ground of the charge for libel, but that had been abandoned; and now it was brought forward to prove a case of conspiracy; but all that that letter did was to say, "You owe 150l., and I request you to pay me." The jury could not shut their eyes to the fact that this was an attempt to convict these men merely by sheer force of prejudice. The jury were asked to say that Wray was a bad fellow, and was trading with inexperienced people, and inducing them to pay him large sums of money. With regard to the charge of threatening to publish a libel, the only letter which could be said to contain any such threat was that which formed the subject of the first indictment, and which had gone off upon the point of venue. Justice, however, would not be defeated by that decision, because the parties were still liable to be tried in Hampshire.

Mr. Kemp then addressed the jury on behalf of Anderson, and submitted that there were many circumstances to rebut the idea of a conspiracy. The only way in which he appeared in these proceedings was as a person who was sent down to Captain Clark's quarters to obtain money, and if in writing a letter to that gentleman he couched it in terms that amounted to a threat to extort money, it must be held to be his own individual act, and could not, therefore, be made the ground of a charge of conspiracy.

Mr. Baron Bramwell summed up the evidence and called the attention of the jury to the letter written by Anderson to Captain Clark on the 5th of

October, from Warburton's Hotel, Newport, and which he described to be clearly an attempt to extort money by threats of exposure. Now, the question was, in what way did the prosecution connect the other prisoner Wray or Henery with this threat made by Anderson, so as to constitute the offence of conspiracy ? There was the letter of the 26th of September from Henery to Captain Clark, in which he referred to Anderson having called upon the prosecutor and demanded 150*l.*, as being due to him (Henery), and then in the same letter he informed the prosecutor that his claim on him was for 150*l.* Then came the letter of the 30th of September addressed to Henery by the Solicitor of Captain Clark, and the receipt of which was acknowledged —not by Henery, but by Anderson, in his letter of the 5th of October, thus showing that there must have been some communication between the two on the subject of the demand made upon Captain Clark. If the jury were satisfied that there was an intent to extort money, by means of threats, and that that intent existed, not only in the mind of one of the prisoners, but in the minds of both, and that they were engaged and leagued together in that common intent, that would amount to a conspiracy, and the prosecutor had made out his case. If they were not so satisfied they would acquit them : but it would certainly be a very singular thing if two people could be found acting in the way in which the prisoners had been acting without some common purpose.

The jury, after a few minutes deliberation, returned a verdict of *Guilty* as against both prisoners.

Mr. Baron BRANWELL in passing sentence, said the offence of which they had been convicted was one of the most abominable that could be conceived. because in a case of this description it was not one robbery that was practised upon the individual who was the subject of it, but that was followed up by a succession of demands until his life was made positively hateful to him. The offence of which they had been found guilty being one of misdemeanor he could not sentence them to more than two years' imprisonment, and he sentenced each of them to be imprisoned for that term, accordingly, with hard labor.

CATALOGUE

OF

MEDICAL, DENTAL,

AND

SCIENTIFIC BOOKS

PUBLISHED BY

LINDSAY & BLAKISTON,

INCLUDING MANY OF THE WORKS ISSUED BY

J. AND A. CHURCHILL, OF LONDON.

All of which are for sale by Booksellers generally, any of which will be sent by mail, postage paid, on the receipt of the retail price, or by Express, C. O. D.

☞ Special Attention given to Filling all Orders.

☞ Catalogues furnished on application.

LINDSAY & BLAKISTON,

MEDICAL PUBLISHERS,

25 South Sixth St.,

Jan. 1, 1880.   PHILADELPHIA.

Medical Text-Books and Works of Reference,

PUBLISHED BY

LINDSAY & BLAKISTON, PHILADELPHIA.

For Sale by all Booksellers or mailed FREE on receipt of price.

———— •◄►• ————

Roberts's Hand-Book of the Practice of Medicine. Uniformly commended by the Profession and the Press. Octavo Price, bound in cloth, $5.00; leather, $6.00.

Trousseau's Clinical Medicine. Complete in two volumes, octavo. Price, in cloth, $8.00; leather, $10.00.

Aitken's Science and Practice of Medicine. Third American, from the Sixth London Edition. Two volumes, royal octavo. Price, in cloth, $12.00; leather, $14.00.

Sanderson's Hand-Book for the Physiological Laboratory. Exercises for Students in Physiology and Histology. 353 Illustrations. Price, in one volume, cloth, $6.00; leather, $7.00.

Cazeaux's Text-Book of Obstetrics. From the Seventh French Edition, Revised and greatly Enlarged. With Illustrations. Cloth, $6.00; leather, $7.00.

Waring's Practical Therapeutics. From the Third London Edition. Cloth, $4.00; leather, $5.00.

Rindfleisch's Pathological Histology. Containing 208 elaborately executed Microscopical Illustrations. Cloth, $5.00; leather, $6.00.

Meigs and Pepper's Practical Treatise on the Diseases of Children. Sixth Edition. Cloth, $6.00; leather, $7.00.

Tanner's Practice of Medicine. The Sixth American Edition, Revised and Enlarged. Cloth, $6.00; leather, $7.00.

Tanner and Meadow's Diseases of Infancy and Childhood. Third Edition. Cloth, $3.00.

Biddle's Materia Medica for Students. The Eighth Revised and Enlarged Edition. With Illustrations. Price, $4.00.

Harris's Principles and Practice of Dentistry. The Tenth Revised and Enlarged Edition. Cloth, $6.50; leather, $7.50.

Soelberg Wells on Diseases of the Eye. Fourth London Edition. Illustrated by Ophthalmoscopic Plates and other Engravings. Cloth, leather.

Woodman and Tidy's Forensic Medicine and Toxicology. Illustrated. 8vo. Cloth, $7.50; sheep, $8.50.

Byford on the Uterus. A New, Enlarged, and thoroughly Revised Edition. Numerous Illustrations Price, $5.00.

Hewitt's Diagnosis and Treatment of the Diseases of Women. Third Edition. Cloth, $4.00; leather, $5.00.

Headland on the Action of Medicines. Sixth American Edition. Price, $3.00.

Atthill's Diseases of Women. Fifth Edition. Numerous Illustrations. Price, $2.25.

Meadow's Manual of Midwifery. Illustrated. Third Enlarged Edition, including the Signs and Symptoms of Pregnancy, etc. Price, $3.00

Bloxom's Chemistry. Inorganic and Organic. Third Edition. 276 Illustrations. Cloth, $4.00; leather, $5.00.

Beale's How to Work with the Microscope. Fifth Edition. 400 Illustrations. $7.50.

Bucknill and Tuke's Psychological Medicine. Fourth Edition. Numerous Illustrations. Price, $8.00.

Wilks and Moxon's Pathological Anatomy. Second Edition, Enlarged and Revised. Price, $6.00

Parke's Manual of Practical Hygiene. The Fifth Enlarged Edition. Price, $6.00.

Fothergill's Complete Manual of the Diseases of the Heart, and their Treatment. Second Edition. Price, $3.50

Bloxam's Laboratory Teaching. Fourth Edition. 80 Illustrations. Price, $1.75.

Taft's Operative Dentistry. Third Edition. 100 Illustrations. Cloth. Price, $4.25.

Wythe's Microscopists' Manual. Third Edition, much Enlarged and Elegantly Illustrated. Price, $2.00

Beale's Use of the Microscope in Practical Medicine. Fourth Edition. 500 Illustrations. Price, $7.50

Sweringen's Dictionary of Pharmaceutical Science. Octavo. Price, $3.00

Mackenzie's Growths in the Larynx With Numerous Colored Illustrations. Price, $2.00.

Tanner's Index of Diseases, and their Treatment. A New Edition Price, $3.00.

Tidy's Hand-Book of Modern Chemistry. Organic and Inorganic. Price, $5.00.

Charteris' Hand-Book of Practice. Illustrated. Price, $2.00.

Fenwick's Outlines of the Practice of Medicine. With special reference to the Prognosis and Treatment of Disease. With Formulæ and Illustrations. Large 12mo Price, $2.00.

THE
Practitioner and Student's Guide Series.

Under this general title the publishers are issuing a New Series of *Medical Text-Books*, or *Hand-Books for Practitioners*, Moderate in Size and Price, and comprising a Series of Treatises on the Elementary and Practical Branches of Medicine. Each one complete in itself. Prepared by Men of Established Reputation. Containing a Condensed Summary of the Existing State of the Science adapted to the wants of all classes of Medical Men. SOLD SEPARATELY.

NOW READY.

1. The Student's Guide to the Practice of Midwifery. By D. LLOYD ROBERTS, M. D., Vice-President of the Obstetrical Society of London, Physician to St. Mary's Hospital, Manchester. With 95 Engravings. Price, $2.00

2. The Student's Guide to the Diseases of Women. With numerous Illustrations. By ALFRED LEWIS GALABIN, M.D., Assistant Obstetric Physician, and Joint Lecturer on Midwifery, Guy's Hospital. 12mo. Cloth......... 2.00

3. The Student's Guide to Dental Anatomy and Surgery. By HENRY E. SEWILL, M. R. C. S. Eng., L. D. S., Dental Surgeon to the West London Hospital. With 77 Engravings..................................... 1.50

4. The Complete Hand-Book of Obstetric Surgery, or, Short Rules of Practice in Every Emergency, from the Simplest to the most Formidable Operations in the Practice of Surgery. By CHARLES CLAY, M. D., Fellow of the London Obstetrical Society, etc. With 101 Illustrations 2.00

5. Surgical Emergencies. A Manual Containing Concise Descriptions of Various Accidents and Emergencies, with Directions for their Immediate Treatment. By W. P. SWAIN, M. D., Surgeon to the Royal Albert Hospital, etc. With 82 Wood Engravings.. 2.00

6. A Manual of Minor Surgery and Bandaging, for the Use of House Surgeons, Dressers, and Junior Practitioners. By CHRISTOPHER HEATH, F. R. C. S., Surgeon to University College Hospital, etc. With a Formulæ and 86 Illustrations 2.00

7. A Hand-Book on the Diseases and Injuries of the Ear. By W. B. DALBY, F. R. C. S., Aural Surgeon to St. George's Hospital. With 21 Illustrations.. 1.50

8. The Student's Hand-Book of the Practice of Medicine. With Microscopic and other Illustrations. By Prof. CHARTERIS, of Glasgow University 2.00

9. Practical Gynæcology. A Hand book for Students and Practitioners. With Illustrations. By HEYWOOD SMITH, M.D., Physician to the Hospital for Women, etc 1.50

A Guide to Surgical Diagnosis. By CHRISTOPHER HEATH, F. R. C. S., Surgeon to University College Hospital, etc. 12mo. Cloth...................... 1 50

Practical Surgery. Including SURGICAL DRESSINGS, BANDAGING LIGATIONS, and AMPUTATIONS. By J. EWING MEARS, M.D., Demonstrator of Surgery in Jefferson Medical College, etc., etc. 227 Illustrations............................. 2.00

Atthill's Clinical Lectures on Diseases Peculiar to Women. Fifth Edition. Revised and Enlarged. With numerous Illustrations............ ...... 2.25

Fenwick's Outlines of the Practice of Medicine. With special reference to the Prognosis and Treatment of Disease. With Formula and Illustrations. Large 12mo.......... ....

LINDSAY & BLAKISTON, Publishers,
25 South Sixth Street, Philadel

ATTHILL (LOMBE), M. D.,

Fellow and Examiner in Midwifery, King and Queen's College of Physicians, Dublin.

CLINICAL LECTURES ON DISEASES PECULIAR TO WO·
MEN. Fifth Edition, Revised and Enlarged, with numerous Illustrations. Price $2.25

The value and popularity of this book is proved by the rapid sale of the first edition,
which was exhausted in less than a year from the time of its publication. It appears to
possess three great merits: First, It treats of the diseases very common to females. Second,
It treats of them in a thoroughly clinical and practical manner. Third, It is concise, original, and illustrated by numerous cases from the author's own experience. His style is clear
and the volume is the result of the author's large and accurate clinical observation recorded
in a remarkable, perspicuous, and terse manner, and is conspicuous for the best qualities of
a practical guide to the student and practitioner. — *British Medical Journal.*

ADAMS (WILLIAM), F. R. C. S.,

Surgeon to the Royal Orthopedic and Great Northern Hospitals.

CLUB-FOOT: ITS CAUSES, PATHOLOGY, AND TREAT-
MENT. Being the Jacksonian Prize Essay of the Royal College of
Surgeons. A New Revised and Enlarged Edition, with 106 Illustrations
engraved on Wood, and Six Lithographic Plates. A large Octavo
Volume. Price $5.00

ADAMS (ROBERT), M. D.,

Regius Professor of Surgery in the University of Dublin, &c., &c.

RHEUMATIC GOUT, OR CHRONIC RHEUMATIC ARTHRI-
TIS OF ALL THE JOINTS. The Second Edition. Illustrated by
numerous Woodcuts, and a quarto Atlas of Plates. 2 Volumes.
Price $7.50

ALTHAUS (JULIUS), M.D.,

Physician to the Infirmary of Epilepsy and Paralysis.

A TREATISE ON MEDICAL ELECTRICITY, Theoretical and
Practical, and its Use in the Treatment of Paralysis, Neuralgia, and other
Diseases. Third Edition, Enlarged and Revised, with One Hundred
and Forty-six Illustrations. In one volume octavo. Price . $6.00

ALLEN (ALFRED H.), F. C. S.,

Lecturer on Chemistry at the Sheffield School of Medicine.

AN INTRODUCTION TO THE PRACTICE OF COMMER-
CIAL ORGANIC ANALYSIS. Being a Treatise on the Properties,
Proximate Analytical Examination, and Modes of Assaying the various
Organic Chemicals and Preparations employed in the Arts, Manufac-
tures, Medicine, etc. ; with Concise Methods for the Detection and
Determination of their Impurities, Adulterations, and Products of De-
composition. Vol. I.—Cyanogen Compounds, Alcohols and their
Derivatives, Phenols, Acids, etc. Price $3.50

AGNEW (D. HAYES), M.D.,

Professor of Surgery in the University of Pennsylvania.

THE LACERATIONS OF THE FEMALE PERINEUM, AND
VESICO-VAGINAL FISTULA, their History and Treatment, with
numerous Illustrations. Octavo. Price $1.50

ACTON (WILLIAM), M.R.C.S., ETC.

THE FUNCTIONS AND DISORDERS OF THE REPRODUC-
TIVE ORGANS. In Childhood, Youth, Adult Age, and Advanced
Life, considered in their Physiological, Social, and Moral Relations.
Fourth American from the Fifth London Edition. Carefully revised by
the Author, with additions. $2.50

Mr. Acton has done good service to society by grappling manfully with sexual vice, and
we trust that others, whose position as men of science and teachers enable them to speak
with authority, will assist in combating and arresting the evils which it entails. The spirit
which pervades his book is one which does credit equally to the head and to the heart of the
author. — *British and Foreign Medico-Chirurgical Review.*

AVELING (J. H.), M. D.,
Physician to Chelsea Hospital for Diseases of Women.

THE INFLUENCE OF POSTURE ON WOMEN IN GYNECIC
AND OBSTETRIC PRACTICE. Octavo. Cloth. Price . $2.00

ANSTIE (FRANCIS E.), M.D.,
Lecturer on Materia Medica and Therapeutics, etc.

STIMULANTS AND NARCOTICS. Their Mutual Relations, with
Special Researches on the Action of Alcohol, Ether, and Chloroform
on the Vital Organism. Octavo. $3.00

ANDERSON (M'CALL), M.D.,
Professor of Clinical Medicine in the University of Glasgow, &c.

ECZEMA. The Pathology and Treatment of the various Eczema-
tous Affections or Eruptions of the Skin. The Third Revised and Enlarged Edition. Octavo. Price $2.50

BUZZARD'S CLINICAL ASPECTS OF SYPHILITIC NER-
VOUS AFFECTIONS. 12mo. Cloth. Price . . . $1.75

BASHAM'S AIDS TO THE DIAGNOSIS OF DISEASES OF
THE KIDNEYS. Sixty Illustrations $1.75

BASHAM ON DROPSY, AND ITS CONNECTION WITH
DISEASES OF THE KIDNEYS, HEART, LUNGS, AND LIVER.
With Sixteen Plates. Third Edition. Octavo . . . $4.50

BARTH AND ROGER'S MANUAL OF AUSCULTATION
AND PERCUSSION. From the Sixth French Edition . $1.00

BRADLEY'S MANUAL OF COMPARATIVE ANATOMY
AND PHYSIOLOGY. Sixty Illustrations. Third Edition . $2.00

BERNAY'S (ALBERT J.), Ph. D.
Professor of Chemistry at St. Thomas's Hospital.

NOTES FOR STUDENTS IN CHEMISTRY. Compiled from
Fowne's and other Manuals. The Sixth Edition. Cloth . $1.25

BY SAME AUTHOR.

THE STUDENT'S GUIDE TO MEDICAL CHEMISTRY.
With Illustrations. Preparing.

BENNETT (J. HENRY), M. D.

NUTRITION IN HEALTH AND DISEASE. A Contribution to Hygiene and to Clinical Medicine. Third Edition, Revised and Enlarged. Octavo. Cloth. Price $2.50

BY SAME AUTHOR.

THE TREATMENT OF PULMONARY CONSUMPTION BY HYGIENE, CLIMATE, AND MEDICINE. With an Appendix on the Sanitaria of the United States, Switzerland, and the Balearic Islands. The Third Edition, much Enlarged. Octavo. Price . $2.50

BUCKNILL (JOHN CHARLES), M.D., & TUKE (DANIEL H.), M.D.

A MANUAL OF PSYCHOLOGICAL MEDICINE: containing the Lunacy Laws, the Nosology, Œtiology, Statistics, Description, Diagnosis, Pathology (including Morbid Histology), and Treatment of Insanity. Fourth Edition, much enlarged, with Twelve Lithographic Plates, and numerous Illustrations. Octavo. Price $8.00

This edition will contain a number of pages of additional matter, and, in consequence of recent advances in Psychological Medicine, several chapters will be rewritten, bringing the Classification, Pathology, and Treatment of Insanity up to the present time.

BURNETT (CHARLES H.), M. D.,
Aurist to the Presbyterian Hospital, &c.

HEARING, AND HOW TO KEEP IT. (Vol. I., American Health Primers.) With Illustrations. Cloth. Price . . . $0.50

BIDDLE (JOHN B.), M. D.,
Professor of Materia Medica and Therapeutics in the Jefferson Medical College, Philadelphia, &c.

MATERIA MEDICA, FOR THE USE OF STUDENTS. With Illustrations. Eighth Edition, Revised and Enlarged. Price $4.00

This new and thoroughly revised edition of Professor Biddle's work has incorporated in it all the improvements as adopted by the New United States Pharmacopœia just issued. It is designed to present the leading facts and principles usually comprised under this head as set forth by the standard authorities, and to fill a vacuum which seems to exist in the want of an elementary work on the subject. The larger works usually recommended as text-books in our Medical schools are too voluminous for convenient use. This will be found to contain, in a condensed form, all that is most valuable, and will supply students with a reliable guide to the course of lectures on Materia Medica as delivered at the various Medical schools in the United States.

BALFOUR (G. W.), M. D.,
Physician to the Royal Infirmary, Edinburgh; Lecturer on Clinical Medicine, &c.

CLINICAL LECTURES ON DISEASES OF THE HEART AND AORTA. With Illustrations. Octavo. Price . . . $4.00

BYFORD (W. H.), A.M., M.D.,
Professor of Obstetrics and Diseases of Women and Children in the Chicago Medical College, &c.

PRACTICE OF MEDICINE AND SURGERY. Applied to the Diseases and Accidents incident to Women. Second Edition, Revised and Enlarged. Octavo. Price

SAME AUTHOR.

ON THE CHRONIC INFLAMMATION AND DISPLACEMENT OF THE UNIMPREGNATED UTERUS. A New, Enlarged, and Thoroughly Revised Edition, with Numerous Illustrations. 8vo. $2.50

Dr. Byford writes the exact present state of medical knowledge on the subjects presented; and does this so clearly, so concisely, so truthfully, and so completely, that his book on the uterus will always meet the approval of the profession, and be everywhere regarded as a popular standard work. — *Buffalo Medical and Surgical Journal.*

BLACK (D. CAMPBELL), M. D.,

L. R. C. S. Edinburgh, Member of the General Council of the University of Glasgow, &c., &c.

THE FUNCTIONAL DISEASES OF THE RENAL, URINARY, and Reproductive Organs, with a General View of Urinary Pathology. Price $2.00

The style of the author is clear, easy, and agreeable, . . . his work is a valuable contribution to medical science, and being penned in that disposition of unprejudiced philosophical inquiry which should always guide a true physician, admirably embodies the spirit of its opening quotation from Professor Huxley.—*Philada. Med. Times.*

BY SAME AUTHOR.

LECTURES ON BRIGHT'S DISEASE OF THE KIDNEYS. Delivered at the Royal Infirmary of Glasgow. With 20 Illustrations, engraved on Wood. One volume, octavo, in Cloth. Price . $1.50

BENTLEY AND TRIMEN'S

MEDICINAL PLANTS. A New Illustrated Work, now Publishing in Monthly Parts. Forty-one Parts Now Ready. Eight Colored Plates in each Part. Price, each, ... $2.00

This work includes full botanical descriptions, and an account of the properties and uses of the principal plants employed in medicine, especial attention being paid to those which are officinal in the British and United States Pharmacopœias. The plants which supply food and substances required by the sick and convalescent will be also included. Each species will be illustrated by a colored plate drawn from nature.

BEASLEY (HENRY).

THE BOOK OF PRESCRIPTIONS. Containing over 3000 Prescriptions, collected from the Practice of the most Eminent Physicians and Surgeons—English, French, and American; comprising also a Compendious History of the Materia Medica, Lists of the Doses of all Officinal and Established Preparations, and an Index of Diseases and their Remedies. Fifth Edition, Revised and Enlarged. Price $2.25

BY SAME AUTHOR.

THE POCKET FORMULARY: A Synopsis of the British and Foreign Pharmacopœias. Tenth Revised Edition. Price . $2.25

THE DRUGGIST'S GENERAL RECEIPT BOOK AND VETERINARY FORMULARY. Eighth Edition. Just Ready. Price, $2.25

BIRCH (S. B.), M. D.,

Member of the Royal Colleg · of Physicians &c.

CONSTIPATED BOWELS; the Various Causes and the Different Means of Cure. Third Edition. Price $1.00

BRAUNE—BELLAMY.

AN ATLAS OF TOPOGRAPHICAL ANATOMY. After Plane Sections of Frozen Bodies, containing Thirty-four Full-page Photographic Plates and numerous other Illustrations on Wood. By WILHELM BRAUNE, Professor of Anatomy in the University of Leipzig. Translated and Edited by EDWARD BELLAMY, F. R. C. S., Senior Assistant Surgeon to, and Lecturer on Anatomy and Teacher of Operative Surgery at, the Charing Cross Hospital, London. A large quarto volume. Price in cloth, $12.00; half morocco, ... $14.00

COHEN (I. SOLIS), M.D.

Lecturer on Laryngoscopy and Diseases of the Throat and Chest in Jefferson Medical College.

ON INHALATION. ITS THERAPEUTICS AND PRACTICE. Including a Description of the Apparatus employed, &c. With Cases and Illustrations. A New Enlarged Edition. Price . . $2.50

SAME AUTHOR.

CROUP. In its Relations to Tracheotomy. Price . . $1.00

CARSON (JOSEPH), M.D.,

Professor of Materia Medica and Pharmacy in the University.

A HISTORY OF THE MEDICAL DEPARTMENT OF THE UNIVERSITY OF PENNSYLVANIA, from its Foundation in 1765: with Sketches of Deceased Professors, &c. $2.00

CHARTERIS (MATHEW), M.D.,

Member of Hospital Staff and Professor in University of Glasgow.

STUDENTS' HAND-BOOK OF THE PRACTICE OF MEDI-CINE. With Microscopic and other Illustrations. Price . $2.00

This book forms one volume of the Students' Guide Series, or Text-Books, now in course of publication.

CARPENTER (W. B.), M.D., F.R.S.

THE MICROSCOPE AND ITS REVELATIONS. The Sixth London Edition, Revised and Enlarged, with more than 500 Illustrations. . . . .

CORR (L. H.), M.D.

OBSTETRIC CATECHISM, or Obstetrics reduced to Questions and Answers. With Numerous Illustrations. Price . . $2.00

CHAVASSE (P. HENRY), F.R.C.S.,

Author of Advice to a Wife, Advice to a Mother, &c.

APHORISMS ON THE MENTAL CULTURE AND TRAIN-ING OF A CHILD, and on various other subjects relating to Health and Happiness. Addressed to Parents. Price . . . $1.00

Dr. Chavasse's works have been very favorably received and had a large circulation, the value of his advice to WIVES and MOTHERS having thus been very generally recognized. This book is a sequel or companion to them, and it will be found both valuable and important to all who have the care of families, and who want to bring up their children to become useful men and women. It is full of fresh thoughts and graceful illustrations.

CLARKE (W. FAIRLIE), M.D.,

Assistant Surgeon to Charing Cross Hospital.

CLARKE'S TREATISE ON DISEASES OF THE TONGUE. With Lithographic and Wood-cut Illustrations. Octavo. Price $4.50

It contains The Anatomy and Physiology of the Tongue, Importance of its Minute Examination, Its Congenital Defects, Atrophy, Hypertrophy, Parasitic Diseases, Inflammation, Syphilis and its effects, Various Tumors to which it is subject, Accidents, Injuries, &c., &c.

COOPER (S.).

A DICTIONARY OF PRACTICAL SURGERY AND ENCY-CLOPÆDIA OF SURGICAL SCIENCE. New Edition, brought down to the present time. By SAMUEL A. LANE, F.R.C.S., assisted by other eminent Surgeons. In two vols., of over 1000 pages each. $10.00

CLAY (CHARLES), M. D.
Fellow of the London Obstetrical Society, &c.

THE COMPLETE HAND-BOOK OF OBSTETRIC SURGERY, or, Short Rules of Practice in Every Emergency, from the Simplest to the most Formidable Operations in the Practice of Surgery. First American from the Third London Edition. With numerous Illustrations. In one volume. $2.00

CHAMBERS (THOMAS K.), M. D.,

LECTURES, CHIEFLY CLINICAL. Illustrative of a Restorative System of Medicine.

CORMACK (SIR JOHN ROSE), K. B., F. R.'S. E., M. D.
Edinburgh and Paris, Fellow Royal College of Physicians, Physician to the Hertford British Hospital, Paris, &c.

CLINICAL STUDIES, Illustrated by Cases observed in Hospital and Private Practice. With Illustrative Plates. 2 Volumes. Octavo. $5.00

COBBOLD (T. SPENCER), M. D., F. R. S.

PARASITES: A Treatise on the Entozoa of Man and Animals; including some Account of the Ectozoa. With 85 Engravings. Octavo. Price $5.00

CLEAVELAND (C. H.), M. D.,
Member of the American Medical Association, &c.

A PRONOUNCING MEDICAL LEXICON. Containing the Correct Pronunciation and Definition of Terms used in Medicine and the Collateral Sciences. Improved Edition, Cloth, 75 cts. ; Tucks, $1.00

This work is not only a Lexicon of all the words in common use in Medicine, but it is also a Pronouncing Dictionary, a feature of great value to Medical Students. To the Dispenser it will prove an excellent aid, and also to the Pharmaceutical Student. It has received strong commendation both from the Medical Press and from the profession.

COLES (OAKLEY), D. D. S.
Dental Surgeon to the Hospital for Diseases of the Throat, &c.

A MANUAL OF DENTAL MECHANICS. Containing much information of a Practical Nature for Practitioners and Students.
INCLUDING

The Preparation of the Mouth for Artificial Teeth, on Taking Impressions, Various Modes of Applying Heat in the Laboratory, Casting in Plaster of Paris and Metal, Precious Metals used in Dentistry, Making Gold Plates, Various Forms of Porcelain used in Mechanical Dentistry, Pivot Teeth, Choosing and Adjusting Mineral Teeth, the Vulcanite Base, the Celluloid Base, Treatment of Deformities of the Mouth, Receipts for Making Gold Plate and Solder, etc., etc.

With 140 Illustrations. Price $2.00

SAME AUTHOR.

ON DEFORMITIES OF THE MOUTH, CONGENITAL AND ACQUIRED, with their Mechanical Treatment. Second Edition, Revised and Enlarged. With Illustrations. Price, . . .

DOMVILLE (EDWARD J.), M. D.

A MANUAL FOR HOSPITAL NURSES and Others engaged in Attending the Sick. 12mo. Price $1.00

CLARK (F. LE GROS), F. R. S.,
Senior Surgeon to St. Thomas's Hospital.

OUTLINES OF SURGERY AND SURGICAL PATHOLOGY,
including the Diagnosis and Treatment of Obscure and Urgent Cases,
and the Surgical Anatomy of some Important Structures and Regions.
Assisted by W. W. WAGSTAFFE, F. R. C. S., Resident Assistant-Surgeon
of, and Joint Lecturer on Anatomy at, St. Thomas's Hospital. Second
Edition, Revised and Enlarged. Price $2.00

COTTLE (E. WYNDHAM), M. A., F. R. C. S., &c.

THE HAIR IN HEALTH AND DISEASE. Partly from Notes
by the late GEORGE NAYLER, F. R. C. S., Surgeon to the Hospital for
Diseases of the Skin, &c. 18mo. Cloth. Price . . $0.75

CURLING (T. B.), F. R. S.,
Consulting Surgeon to the London Hospital, &c.

A PRACTICAL TREATISE ON THE DISEASES OF THE
TESTIS AND OF THE SPERMATIC CORD AND SCROTUM.
Fourth Revised and Enlarged Edition. Octavo. Price. . $5.50

BY SAME AUTHOR.

OBSERVATIONS ON DISEASES OF THE RECTUM. With
Illustrations. Fourth Edition, Revised and Enlarged. Octavo. Cloth.
Price $2.75

CAZEAUX (P.), M. D.,
Adjunct Professor of the Faculty of Medicine, Paris, etc.

A THEORETICAL AND PRACTICAL TREATISE ON MIDWIFERY,
including the Diseases of Pregnancy and Parturition. Translated from
the Seventh French Edition, Revised, Greatly Enlarged, and Improved,
by S. TARNIER, Clinical Chief of the Lying-In Hospital, Paris, etc.,
with numerous Lithographic and other Illustrations. Price, in Cloth,
$6.00 ; in Leather $7.00

M. Cazeaux's Great Work on Obstetrics has become classical in its character, and almost
an Encyclopædia in its fulness. Written expressly for the use of students of medicine, its
teachings are plain and explicit, presenting a condensed summary of the leading principles
established by the masters of the obstetric art, and such clear, practical directions for the
management of the pregnant, parturient, and puerperal states, as have been sanctioned by
the most authoritative practitioners, and confirmed by the author's own experience.

DOBELL (HORACE), M. D.,
Senior Physician to the Hospital.

WINTER COUGH (CATARRH, BRONCHITIS, EMPHYSEMA,
ASTHMA). Lectures Delivered at the Royal Hospital for Diseases of
the Chest. The Third Enlarged Edition, with Colored Plates. Octavo.
Price $3.50

BY SAME AUTHOR.

ON LOSS OF WEIGHT, BLOOD-SPITTING, AND LUNG
DISEASE. With a Colored Frontispiece of the Lung, a Tabular Map,
&c., &c. Octavo. Cloth. Price . . . . . $3.25.

DIXON (JAMES), F. R. C. S.

Surgeon to the Royal London Ophthalmic Hospital, &c.

A GUIDE TO THE PRACTICAL STUDY OF DISEASES OF
THE EYE, with an Outline of their Medical and Operative Treatment,
with Test Types and Illustrations. Third Edition, thoroughly Revised,
and a great portion Rewritten. Price $2.00

Mr. Dixon's book is essentially a practical one, written by an observant author, who brings
to his special subject a sound knowledge of general Medicine and Surgery.—*Dublin Quarterly.*

DILLNBERGER (DR. EMIL).

A HANDY-BOOK OF THE TREATMENT OF WOMEN AND
CHILDREN'S DISEASES, according to the Vienna Medical School.
Part I. The Diseases of Women. Part II. The Diseases of Children.
Translated from the Second German Edition, by P. NICOL, M. D.
Price $1.50

Many practitioners will be glad to possess this little manual, which gives a large mass
of practical hints on the treatment of diseases which probably make up the larger half of
every-day practice. The translation is well made, and explanations of reference to German
medicinal preparations are given with proper fulness. — *The Practitioner.*

DUNGLISON (RICHARD J.), M. D.

THE PRACTITIONER'S REFERENCE BOOK. Containing
Therapeutic and Practical Hints, Dietetic Rules and Precepts, and
other General Information Useful to the Physician, Pharmacist, and
Student. Octavo. Cloth. Price $3.50

DUCHENNE (DR. G. B.).

LOCALIZED ELECTRIZATION AND ITS APPLICATION
TO PATHOLOGY AND THERAPEUTICS. Translated by HER-
BERT TIBBITS, M. D. With Ninety-two Illustrations. Price . $3.00

Duchenne's great work is not only a well-nigh exhaustive treatise on the medical uses of
Electricity, but it is also an elaborate exposition of the different diseases in which Electricity has proved to be of value as a therapeutic and diagnostic agent.

PART II., illustrated by chromo-lithographs and numerous wood-cuts, is preparing.

DURKEE (SILAS), M. D.,

Fellow of the Massachusetts Medical Society, &c.

GONORRHŒA AND SYPHILIS. The Sixth Edition, Revised
and Enlarged, with Portraits and Eight Colored Illustrations. Octavo.
Price $3.50

Dr. Durkee's work impresses the reader in favor of the author by its general tone, the
thorough honesty everywhere evinced, the skill with which the book is arranged, the manner in which the facts are cited, the clever way in which the author's experience is brought
in, the lucidity of the reasoning, and the care with which the therapeutics of venereal complaints are treated. — *Lancet.*

DRUITT (ROBERT), F.R.C.S.

THE SURGEON'S VADE-MECUM. A Manual of Modern Surgery. The Eleventh Revised and Enlarged Edition, with 369 Illustrations. Price $5.00

DALBY (w. b.), F. R. C. S.,

Aural Surgeon to St. George's Hospital.

LECTURES ON THE DISEASES AND INJURIES OF THE EAR. Delivered at St. George's Hospital. With Illustrations. Price $1.50

We cordially recommend this admirable volume by Mr. Dalby as a trustworthy guide in the treatment of the affections of the ear. The book is moderate in price, beautifully illus-trated by wood-cuts, and got up in the best style. — *Glasgow Medical Journal.*

DAY (WILLIAM HENRY), M. D.,

Physician to the Samaritan Hospital for Women and Children, &c.

HEADACHES, THEIR NATURE, CAUSES, AND TREAT-MENT. Second Edition. 12mo. Cloth. Price . . $2.00

ELLIS (EDWARD), M. D.,

Physician to the Victoria Hospital for Sick Children, &c.

A PRACTICAL MANUAL OF THE DISEASES OF CHIL-DREN, with a Formulary. Third Enlarged Edition, Revised and Improved. One volume $2.50

The AUTHOR, in issuing this new edition of his book, says: " I have very carefully revised each chapter, adding several new sections, and making considerable additions where the subjects seemed to require fuller treatment, without, however, sacrificing conciseness or unduly increasing the bulk of the volume."

FENWICK (SAMUEL).

OUTLINES OF THE PRACTICE OF MEDICINE. With special reference to the Prognosis and Treatment of Disease. With Formula and Illustrations. Large 12mo. Price $2.00

FOTHERGILL (J. MILNER), M. D.,

Assistant Physician to City of London Hospital for Diseases of the Chest, &c.

THE HEART, ITS DISEASES AND THEIR TREATMENT, including the Gouty Heart. Second Edition, Entirely Rewritten and Enlarged, with Two Full-Page Lithographic Plates and Forty other Illustrations. Octavo. Price $3.50

" Dr. Fothergill's remarks on rest, on proper blood nutrition in Heart Disease, in the treatment of Sequelæ of it, and on the action of special medicines, all indicate that in study-ing the pathology of Heart Disease, he has earnestly kept in view the best means of mitigat-ing suffering and of prolonging life." — *Lancet.*

FOX (CORNELIUS B.), M. D.

SANITARY EXAMINATIONS of Water, Air, and Food. 94 En-gravings. 8vo. Price $4.00

FOX (TILBURY), M. D., F. R. C. P.

Physician to the Department for Skin Diseases in University College Hospital.

ATLAS OF SKIN DISEASES. Consisting of a Series of Colored Illustrations, in Monthly Parts, together with Descriptive Text and Notes upon Treatment ; each Part containing Four Plates, reproduced by Chromo-Lithography from the work of Willan & Bateman, or taken from Original Sources. Now Complete in 18 Parts. Price, per Part, $2.00 ; or in one large Folio volume, bound in cloth. Price . . $30.00

FENNER (c. s.), M. D., &c.

VISION: ITS OPTICAL DEFECTS, and the Adaptation of Spectacles; embracing Physical Optics, Physiological Optics, Errors of Refraction and Defects of Accommodation, or Optical Defects of the Eye. With 74 Illustrations. Selections from the Test Types of Jaeger and Snellen, etc. Octavo. Price $3.50

FOSTER (BALTHAZAR), M.D.,
Professor of Medicine in Queen's College.

LECTURES AND ESSAYS ON CLINICAL MEDICINE. Revised and Enlarged by the Author. With Engravings. Octavo. Price $3.00

FRANKLAND (E.), M. D., F. R. S., &c.

HOW TO TEACH CHEMISTRY, being the substance of Six Lectures to Science Teachers. Reported, with the Author's sanction, by G. George Chaloner, F. C. S., &c. With Illustrations . $1.25

FULTON (J.), M. D.,
Professor of Physiology, Trinity Medical College, Toronto.

A TEXT-BOOK OF PHYSIOLOGY. Second Edition, Revised and Enlarged. With numerous Illustrations. Octavo. Price $4.00

FLINT (AUSTIN), M. D.,
Professor of the Principles and Practice of Medicine, &c., Bellevue Hospital College, New York.

CLINICAL REPORTS ON CONTINUED FEVER. Based on an Analysis of One Hundred and Sixty-four Cases, with Remarks on the Management of Continued Fever; the Identity of Typhus and Typhoid Fever; Diagnosis, &c., &c. Octavo. Price . . $2.00

GANT (FREDERICK J.), F. R. C. S.,
Assisted by Drs. Morrell Mackenzie, Barnes, Erasmus Wilson, and other Specialists.

THE SCIENCE AND PRACTICE OF SURGERY. Second Edition. 1700 Pages. 1000 Illustrations. 2 Vols. Price, cloth, $11.00; sheep $13.00

DISEASES OF THE BLADDER, PROSTATE GLAND, AND URETHRA, including a Practical View of Urinary Diseases, Deposits, and Calculi. Fourth Edition, Revised and Enlarged. With New Illustrations. Now Ready. Price $3.50

GODLEE (R. J.), M. D.,
Assistant-Surgeon University College Hospital.

AN ATLAS OF HUMAN ANATOMY. Illustrating the Anatomy of the Human Body, in a Series of Dissections. Accompanied by References and an Explanatory Text. To be completed in Twelve or Thirteen Bi-monthly Parts, Folio Size, each Part containing Four large Colored Plates, or Eight Figures. Ten Parts Now Ready. Price per Part $2.50

GROSS (SAMUEL D.), M. D.,
Professor of Surgery in the Jefferson Medical College, Philadelphia, etc.

AMERICAN MEDICAL BIOGRAPHY OF THE NINETEENTH CENTURY. With a Portrait of BENJAMIN RUSH, M.D. Octavo. $3.50

GREENHOW (E. HEADLAM), M. D.,
Fellow of the Royal College of Physicians, etc.

ON CHRONIC BRONCHITIS, Especially as Connected with Gout, Emphysema, and Diseases of the Heart. Price . . . $1.50

ADDISON'S DISEASE. Illustrated by numerous Cases and 5 full-page Colored Engravings. Price $3.00

GOWERS (W. R.), M. D., F. R. C. P.,
Assistant Professor of Clinical Medicine in University College.

A MANUAL AND ATLAS OF MEDICAL OPHTHALMO-SCOPY. With 16 Colored, Autotype, and Lithographic Plates, and 26 Woodcuts, comprising 112 original Illustrations of the Changes in the Eye in Diseases of the Brain, Kidneys, etc. Octavo. . . $6.00

GALLABIN (ALFRED LEWIS), M. D.,
Assistant Obstetric Physician and Joint Lecturer on Midwifery, Guy's Hospital, &c.

THE STUDENT'S GUIDE TO THE DISEASES OF WOMEN. With Numerous Illustrations. 12mo. Cloth. Price . . $2.00

HIGGINS (CHARLES), F. R. C. S.,
Ophthalmic Surgeon, Guy's Hospital, &c.

HINTS ON OPHTHALMIC OUT-PATIENT PRACTICE. Second Edition. 16mo. Cloth. Price . . . . 60 cts.

HUNTER (CHARLES).
MECHANICAL DENTISTRY. A Practical Treatise on the Construction of the Various Kinds of Artificial Dentures, with Formulæ, Receipts, &c. 100 Illustrations. Price $2.25

HEATH (CHRISTOPHER), F. R. C. S.,
Surgeon to University College Hospital and Holme Professor of Clinical Surgery in University College.

OPERATIVE SURGERY. Elegantly Illustrated by 20 Large Colored Plates, Imperial Quarto Size, each Plate containing several Figures, drawn from Nature by M. Léveillé, of Paris, and Colored by hand under his direction. Complete in Five Quarterly Parts. Price, per Part, $2.50; or in one volume, handsomely bound in cloth. Price $14.00

HEWITT (GRAILY), M. D.,
Physician to the British Lying-in Hospital, and Lecturer on Diseases of Women and Children, &c.

THE DIAGNOSIS, PATHOLOGY, AND TREATMENT OF DISEASES OF WOMEN, including the Diagnosis of Pregnancy. Founded on a Course of Lectures delivered at St. Mary's Hospital Medical School. The Third Edition, Revised and Enlarged, with new Illustrations. Octavo. Price in Cloth . . . $4.00
" Leather . . . 5.00

This new edition of Dr. Hewitt's book has been so much modified, that it may be considered substantially a new book; very much of the matter has been entirely rewritten, and the whole work has been rearranged in such a manner as to present a most decided improvement over previous editions. Dr. Hewitt is the leading clinical teacher on Diseases of Women in London, and the characteristic attention paid to Diagnosis by him has given his work great popularity.

HARDWICH AND DAWSON.

HARDWICH'S MANUAL OF PHOTOGRAPHIC CHEMISTRY.
With Engravings. Eighth Edition. Edited and Rearranged by G.
Dawson, Lecturer on Photography, &c., &c. 12mo . . $2.00

HARLAN (george c.), M. D.,
Surgeon to Wills' Eye Hospital, &c.

EYESIGHT, AND HOW TO CARE FOR IT. (Vol. IV., American Health Primers.) Cloth. Price $0.50

HEADLAND (f. w.), M. D.,
Fellow of the Royal College of Physicians, &c., &c,

ON THE ACTION OF MEDICINES IN THE SYSTEM. Sixth
American from the Fourth London Edition. Revised and Enlarged.
Octavo. Price $3.00

Dr. Headland's work gives the only scientific and satisfactory view of the action of medicine; and this not in the way of idle speculation, but by demonstration and experiments,
and inferences almost as indisputable as demonstrations. It is truly a great scientific work
in a small compass, and deserves to be the hand-book of every lover of the Profession. It
has received the approbation of the *Medical Press*, both in this country and in Europe, and
is pronounced by them to be the most *original* and practically useful work that has been
issued for many years.

HOFF (o.), M. D.

ON HÆMATURIA as a Symptom of Diseases of the Genito-Urinary Organs. Illustrated. 12mo. Cloth. $0.75

HEATH (christopher), F.R.C.S.,
Surgeon to University College Hospital, &c.

INJURIES AND DISEASES OF THE JAWS. The Jacksonian
Prize Essay of the Royal College of Surgeons of England, 1867. Second Edition, Revised, with over 150 Illustrations. Octavo. Price,
$4.25

SAME AUTHOR.

A MANUAL OF MINOR SURGERY AND BANDAGING, for
the Use of House Surgeons, Dressers, and Junior Practitioners. With
a Formulæ and Numerous Illustrations. 16mo. Price . $2.00

A GUIDE TO SURGICAL DIAGNOSIS, for Practitioners and
Students. 12mo. Cloth. Price $1.50

HAYDEN (thomas), M. D.,
Fellow of the King and Queen's College of Physicians, &c., &c.

THE DISEASES OF THE HEART AND AORTA. With 8r
Illustrations. In two volumes, Octavo, of over 1200 pages. Price, $6.00

HUFELAND (c. w.), M. D.

THE ART OF PROLONGING LIFE. Edited by Erasmus Wilson, M. D., F. R. S., &c. 12mo. Cloth. $1.00

HAY (thomas), M. D.,

HISTORY OF A CASE OF RECURRING SARCOMATOUS
TUMOUR OF THE ORBIT IN A CHILD. With Three Full Page
Illustrations, representing the Tumour in its Various Stages. Price, $0.50

JAMES (PROSSER), M. D., M. R. C. P.,
Physician to Throat Hospital.

SORE THROAT: Its Nature, Varieties, and Treatment, and its Connection with other Diseases. Fourth Edition. Colored Plates. 12mo.
Price $2.00

JONES' AURAL ATLAS.

AN ATLAS OF DISEASES OF THE MEMBRANA TYMPANI.
Being a Series of Colored Plates, containing 62 Figures. With appropriate Letter-Press and Explanatory Text by H. McNAUGHTON JONES, M.D., Surgeon to the Cork Ophthalmic and Aural Hospital. 4to.
Cloth. Price $6.00

KIDD (JOSEPH), M. D., M. R. C. S. ·

THE LAWS OF THERAPEUTICS, or The Science and Art of Medicine. 12mo. Cloth. Price $1.25

LONGLEY (ELIAS).

Author of a "Pronouncing Vocabulary of Geographical and Personal Names," &c.

STUDENT'S POCKET MEDICAL LEXICON. Giving the Correct Pronunciation and Definition of all Words and Terms in general use in Medicine and the Collateral Sciences. The Pronunciation being plainly represented in the American Phonetic Alphabet. With an Appendix, containing a Complete List of Poisons and their Antidotes, Abbreviations used in Prescriptions, and a Metric Scale of Doses. 24mo. Cloth. Price, $1.00; in Leather, with Tucks and Pocket, $1.25

This is an entirely new Medical Dictionary, containing some 300 compactly printed 24mo pages, very carefully prepared by the author, who has had much experience in the preparation of similar works, assisted by the Professors of Chemistry and of Botany in one of our leading Medical Colleges. It contains all medical terms in common use, with their pronunciation and definition, without being encumbered with obsolete or useless words. It is essentially new in many of its features, and fully brought up to the present state of medical science.

LAWSON (GEORGE), F.R.C.S.,
Surgeon to the Royal London Ophthalmic Hospital.

DISEASES AND INJURIES OF THE EYE, THEIR MEDICAL AND SURGICAL TREATMENT. Containing a Formulary, Test Types, and Numerous Illustrations. Price . . . . . ·

LEBER & ROTTENSTEIN (DRS.).

DENTAL CARIES AND ITS CAUSES. An Investigation into the Influence of Fungi in the destruction of the Teeth, translated by THOMAS H. CHANDLER, D.M.D., Professor of Mechanical Dentistry in the Dental School of Harvard University. With Illustrations. Octavo.
Price $1.25

LEARED (ARTHUR), M. D., F. R. C. P.

IMPERFECT DIGESTION: ITS CAUSES AND TREATMENT.
The Sixth Edition, Revised and Enlarged. $1.50

KOLLMEYER (A. H.), A. M., M. D.
Professor of Materia Medica and Therapeutics, Montreal College.

CHEMIA COARTATA; or, The Key to Modern Chemistry. With Numerous Tables, Tests, &c., &c. Price, ... $2.25

MAUNDER (c. f.), F. R. C. S.

Surgeon to the London Hospital; formerly Demonstrator of Anatomy at Guy's Hospital.

OPERATIVE SURGERY. Second Edition, with One Hundred and Sixty-four Engravings on Wood. Price . . . **$2.25**

BY SAME AUTHOR.

SURGERY OF THE ARTERIES, including Aneurisms, Wounds, Hæmorrhages, Twenty-seven Cases of Ligatures, Antiseptic, etc. With 18 Illustrations. Price **$1.50**

MAYNE (R. G.), M. D., AND MAYNE (J.), M. D.

MEDICAL VOCABULARY: An Explanation of all Names, Synonyms, Terms, and Phrases used in Medicine and the Relative Branches of Medical Science. 4th Edition. 450 pages. Price, **$3.00**

MAYS (THOMAS J.), M. D.

ON THE THERAPEUTIC FORCES. An Effort to Consider the Action of Medicines in the Light of the Doctrine of Conservation of Force. 12mo. Cloth. Price **$1.25**

MARTIN (JOHN H.).

Author of Microscopic Objects, &c.

A MANUAL OF MICROSCOPIC MOUNTING. With Notes on the Collection and Examination of Objects, and upwards of One Hundred and Fifty Illustrations. Second Edition, Enlarged. Price, **$2.75**

MEADOWS (ALFRED), M. D.

Physician to the Hospital for Women, and to the General Lying-In Hospital, &c.

MANUAL OF MIDWIFERY. A New Text-Book. Including the Signs and Symptoms of Pregnancy, Obstetric Operations, Diseases of the Puerperal State, &c., &c. Second American from the Third London Edition. Revised and Enlarged. With 145 Illustrations. **$3.00**

This book is especially valuable to the Student as containing in a condensed form a large amount of valuable information on the subject which it treats. It is also clear and methodical in its arrangement, and therefore useful as a work of reference for the practitioner. The Illustrations are numerous and well executed.

MILLER (JAMES), F. R. C. S.

Professor of Surgery University of Edinburgh.

ALCOHOL, ITS PLACE AND POWER. From the Nineteenth Glasgow Edition. 12mo. Cloth flexible. Price . . . **$0.50**

LIZARS (JOHN), M. D.

THE USE AND ABUSE OF TOBACCO. Price . . **$0.50**

MILLER AND LIZARS.

ALCOHOL: Its Place and Power. By JAMES MILLER, F.R.S.E., late Professor of Surgery in the University of Edinburgh, &c.—THE USE AND ABUSE OF TOBACCO. By JOHN LIZARS, late Professor to the Royal College of Surgeons, &c. The Two Essays in One Volume. 12mo. **$1.00**

MARSDEN (ALEXANDER), M. D.

A NEW AND SUCCESSFUL MODE OF TREATING CERTAIN
FORMS OF CANCER. Second Edition, Colored Plates. . $3.00

MACDONALD (J. D.), M. D.,
Deputy Inspector-General of Hospitals, Assistant Professor of Hygiene, Army Medical School, &c.

A GUIDE TO THE MICROSCOPICAL EXAMINATION OF
DRINKING WATER. With Twenty Full-page Lithographic Plates,
References, Tables, etc., etc. Octavo. Price . . . $2.75

NORRIS (GEORGE W.), M. D.,
Late Surgeon to the Pennsylvania Hospital, &c.

CONTRIBUTIONS TO PRACTICAL SURGERY, including
numerous Clinical Histories, Drawn from a Hospital Service of Thirty
Years. In one Volume, Octavo. Price $4.00

OTT (ISAAC), M. D.,
Late Demonstrator of Experimental Physiology in the University of Pennsylvania.

THE ACTION OF MEDICINES. With Twenty-two Illustrations.
Octavo. Cloth. Price $2.00

OGSTON (FRANCIS AND FRANCIS, JR.), M. D.
Professor of Medical Jurisprudence, and Assistant Professor in the University of Aberdeen.

LECTURES ON MEDICAL JURISPRUDENCE. With Copper-
plate Illustrations. Octavo. Cloth $6.00

PHYSICIAN'S VISITING LIST, PUBLISHED ANNUALLY.

SIZES AND PRICES.

For 25 Patients weekly.		Tucks, pockets, and pencil,		.	.	.	$1.00
50	"	"	"	"	"	.	.	.	1.25
75	"	"	"	"	"	.	.	.	1.50
100	"	"	"	"	"	.	.	.	2.00
50	"	" 2 vols.	{ Jan. to June } { July to Dec. }	"	.	.	.	2.50
100	"	" 2 vols.	{ Jan. to June } { July to Dec. }	"	.	.	.	3.00

INTERLEAVED EDITION.

For 25 Patients weekly, interleaved, tucks, pockets, &c.,				.	.	1.25
50	"	"	"	"	"	"	.	.	1.50
50	"	" 2 vols.	{ Jan. to June } { July to Dec. }	"	"	.	.	3.00

This Visiting List, now in its twenty-ninth year, contains the Metric or French Decimal System of Weights and Measures, a Posological Table with the Doses in both the Apothecaries and Decimal Metric System of Weights and Measures, a new Table of Poisons, etc.

POWER, HOLMES, ANSTIE, AND BARNES.

REPORTS ON THE PROGRESS OF MEDICINE AND SUR-
GERY, PHYSIOLOGY, OPHTHALMIC MEDICINE, MID-
WIFERY, DISEASES OF WOMEN AND CHILDREN, MATERIA
MEDICA, &c. Edited for the Sydenham Society of London. Octavo.
Price $2.00

PARKES (EDWARD A.), M. D., ·
Professor of Military Hygiene in the Army Medical School, &c.

A MANUAL OF PRACTICAL HYGIENE. The Fifth Revised and Enlarged Edition, for Medical Officers of the Army, Civil Medical Officers, Boards of Health, &c., &c. With many Illustrations. One Volume Octavo. Price $6.00

This work, previously unrivalled as a text-book for medical officers of the army, is now equally unrivalled as a text-book for civil medical officers. The first book treats in successive chapters of water, air, ventilation, examination of air, food, quality, choice, and cooking of food, beverages, and condiments; soil, habitations, removal of excreta, warming of houses, exercise, clothing, climate, meteorology, individual hygienic management, disposal of the dead, the prevention of some common diseases, disinfection, and statistics. The second book is devoted to the service of the soldier, but is hardly less instructive to the civil officer of health. It is, in short, a comprehensive and trustworthy text-book of hygiene for the scientific or general reader.— *London Lancet.*

OSGOOD (HAMILTON), M. D.,
Editorial Staff Boston Medical and Surgical Journal.

WINTER AND ITS DANGERS. (Vol. V., American Health Primers.) Cloth. Price $0.50

PENNSYLVANIA HOSPITAL REPORTS.

EDITED BY A COMMITTEE OF THE HOSPITAL STAFF. J. M. Da Costa, M. D., and William Hunt, M. D. Vols. 1 and 2; each volume containing upwards of Twenty Original Articles, by former and present Members of the Staff, now eminent in the Profession, with Lithographic and other Illustrations. Price per volume . $2.00

The first Reports were so favorably received, on both sides of the Atlantic, that it is hardly necessary to speak for them the universal welcome of which they are deserving. The papers are all valuable contributions to the literature of medicine, reflecting great credit upon their authors. The work is one of which the Pennsylvania Hospital may well be proud. It will dô much towards elevating the profession of this country.— *American Journal of Obstetrics.*

PAGET (JAMES), F. R. S.,
Surgeon to St. Bartholomew's Hospital, &c.

SURGICAL PATHOLOGY. Lectures delivered at the Royal College of Surgeons of England. Third London Edition, Edited and Revised by William Turner, M. D. With Numerous Illustrations. Price, in cloth, $7.00; in leather $8.00

A new and revised edition of Mr. Paget's Classical Lectures needs no introduction to our readers. Commendation would be as superfluous as criticism out of place. Every page bears evidence that this edition has been " carefully revised."— *American Medical Journal.*

PEREIRA (JONATHAN), M. D., F. R. S., &c.

PHYSICIAN'S PRESCRIPTION BOOK. Containing Lists of Terms, Phrases, Contractions, and Abbreviations used in Prescriptions, with Explanatory Notes, the Grammatical Constructions of Prescriptions, Rules for the Pronunciation of Pharmaceutical Terms, a Prosodiacal Vocabulary of the Names of Drugs, &c., and a Series of Abbreviated Prescriptions illustrating the use of the preceding terms, &c. ; to which is added a Key, containing the Prescriptions in an unabbreviated Form, with a Literal Translation, intended for the use of Medical and Pharmaceutical Students. From the Fifteenth London Edition. Price, in cloth, * 1.00; in leather, with Tucks and Pocket, . . $1.25

PARSONS (CHARLES), M. D.,

Honorary Surgeon to the Dover Convalescent Homes, &c., &c.

SEA-AIR AND SEA-BATHING. Their Influence on Health a Practical Guide for the Use of Visitors at the Seaside. 18mo. $0.60

PARKER (LANGSTON), F. R. C. S. L.

THE MODERN TREATMENT OF SYPHILITIC DISEASES. Containing the Treatment of Constitutional and Confirmed Syphilis, with numerous Cases, Formulæ,&c.,&c. Fifth Edition,Enlarged. $4.25

PRINCE (DAVID), M. D.

PLASTIC AND ORTHOPEDIC SURGERY. Containing 1. A Report on the Condition of, and Advances made in, Plastic and Orthopedic Surgery up to the Year 1871. 2. A New Classification and Brief Exposition of Plastic Surgery. With numerous Illustrations. 3. Orthopedics: A Systematic Work upon the Prevention and Cure of Deformities. With numerous Illustrations. Octavo. Price . . . $4.50

This is a good book upon an important practical subject; carefully written and abundantly illustrated. It goes over the whole ground of deformities—from cleft-palate and club-foot to spinal curvatures and ununited fractures. It appears, moreover, to be an original book. — *Medical and Surgical Reporter.*

SAME AUTHOR.

GALVANO-THERAPEUTICS. A Revised reprint of A Report made to the Illinois State Medical Society. With Illustrations. Price, $1.25

PIESSE (G. W. SEPTIMUS),

Analytical Chemist.

WHOLE ART OF PERFUMERY. And the Methods of Obtaining the Odors of Plants; the Manufacture of Perfumes for the Handkerchief, Scented Powders, Odorous Vinegars, Dentifrices, Pomatums, Cosmetics, Perfumed Soaps, &c.; the Preparation of Artificial Fruit Essences, &c. Second American from the Third London Edition. With Illustrations. New Edition preparing.

PIGGOTT (A. SNOWDEN), M. D.,

Practical Chemist.

COPPER MINING AND COPPER ORE. Containing a full Description of some of the Principal Copper Mines of the United States, the Art of Mining, the Mode of Preparing the Ore for Market, &c., &c. $1.00

PAVY (F. W.), M. D., F. R. S.

DIABETES. Researches on its Nature and Treatment. Third Revised Edition. Octavo . . . .

PHYSICIAN'S PRESCRIPTION BLANKS, with a Margin for Duplicates, Notes, Cases, &c., &c. Price, per package, .
Price, per dozen . .

RADCLIFFE (CHARLES BLAND), M.D.,
Fellow of the Royal College of Physicians of London, &c.

LECTURES ON EPILEPSY, PAIN, PARALYSIS, and other
Disorders of the Nervous System. With Illustrations. . . $1.50

The reputation which Dr. Radcliffe possesses as a very able authority on nervous affections
will commend his work to every medical practitioner. We recommend it as a work that will
throw much light upon the Physiology and Pathology of the Nervous System. — *Canada
Medical Journal.*

ROBERTSON (A.), M.D., D.D.S.

A MANUAL ON EXTRACTING TEETH. Founded on the
Anatomy of the Parts involved in the Operation, the kinds and proper
construction of the instruments to be used, the accidents likely to occur
from the operation, and the proper remedies to retrieve such accidents.
A New Revised Edition. . . . .

RICHARDSON (JOSEPH G.), M.D.,
Professor of Hygiene in Pennsylvania University.

LONG LIFE, AND HOW TO REACH IT. (Vol. II., American
Health Primers.) Cloth. Price $0.50

REESE (JOHN J.), M.D.,
Professor of Medical Jurisprudence and Toxicology in the University of Pennsylvania.

AN ANALYSIS OF PHYSIOLOGY. Being a Condensed View
of the most important Facts and Doctrines, designed especially for the
Use of Students. Second Edition, Enlarged. . . . $1.50

SAME AUTHOR.

THE AMERICAN MEDICAL FORMULARY. Price . $1.50

A SYLLABUS OF MEDICAL CHEMISTRY. Price . $1.00

RICHARDSON (JOSEPH), D.D.S.
Late Professor of Mechanical Dentistry, &c., &c.

A PRACTICAL TREATISE ON MECHANICAL DENTISTRY.
Second Edition, much Enlarged. With over 150 beautifully executed
Illustrations. Octavo.

This work does infinite credit to its author. Its comprehensive style has in no way interfered with most elaborate details where this is necessary; and the numerous and beautifully
executed wood-cuts with which it is illustrated make the volume as attractive as its instructions are easily understood. —*Edinburgh Med. Journal.*

ROBERTS (LLOYD D.), M.D.,
Vice-President of the Obstetrical Society of London, Physician to St. Mary's Hospital, Manchester.

THE STUDENT'S GUIDE TO THE PRACTICE OF MID-
WIFERY. With 95 Illustrations. Price $2.00

RUTHERFORD (WILLIAM), M.D., F.R.S.E.
Professor of the Institutes of Medicine in the University of Edinburgh.

OUTLINES OF PRACTICAL HISTOLOGY FOR STUDENTS
AND OTHERS. Second Edition, Revised and Enlarged. With Illustrations, &c. Price $2.00

RIGBY and MEADOWS.

DR. RIGBY'S OBSTETRIC MEMORANDA. Fourth Edition, Revised and Enlarged, by ALFRED MEADOWS, M. D., Author of "A Manual of Midwifery," &c. Price **$0.50**

ROYLE'S MANUAL OF MATERIA MEDICA AND THERA-

PEUTICS. The Sixth Revised and Enlarged Edition. Containing all the New Preparations according to the New British, American, French, and German Pharmacopœias, the New Chemical Nomenclature, etc., etc. Edited by JOHN HARLEY, M. D., F. R. C. P., Assistant Physician and Lecturer on Physiology at St. Thomas's Hospital. With 139 Illustrations, many of them new. One vol., Demy Octavo. **$5.00**

STOCKEN (JAMES), L. D. S. R. C. S.,

Lecturer on Dental Materia Medica and Therapeutics and Dental Surgeon to National Dental Hospital.

THE ELEMENTS OF DENTAL MATERIA MEDICA AND THERAPEUTICS. With Pharmacopœia. Second Edition. **$2.25**

SANDERSON, KLEIN, FOSTER, and BRUNTON.

A HAND-BOOK FOR THE PHYSIOLOGICAL LABORATORY. Being Practical Exercises for Students in Physiology and Histology, by E. KLEIN, M. D., Assistant Professor in the Pathological Laboratory of the Brown Institution, London; J. BURDON-SANDERSON, M. D., F. R. S., Professor of Practical Theology in University College, London; MICHAEL FOSTER, M.D., F.R.S., Fellow of and Prælector of Physiology in Trinity College, Cambridge; and T. LAUDER BRUNTON, M.D., D.Sc., Lecturer on Materia Medica in the Medical College of St. Bartholomew's Hospital. Edited by J. BURDON-SANDERSON. The Illustrations consist of One Hundred and Twenty-three octavo pages, including over Three Hundred and Fifty Figures, with appropriate letter-press explanations attached and references to the text. Price, in one volume, Cloth, $6.00; in Leather, $7.00; or in two volumes, Cloth, $7.00. Vol. I., containing the Text, sold separately, $4.00.

We feel that we cannot recommend this work too highly. To those engaged in physiological work as students or teachers, it is almost indispensable; and to those who are not, a perusal of it will by no means be unprofitable. The execution of the plates leaves nothing to be desired. They are mostly original, and their arrangement in a separate volume has great and obvious advantages.— *Dublin Journal of Medical Sciences.*

SIEVEKING (E. H.), M.D., F.R.C.S.

THE MEDICAL ADVISER IN LIFE ASSURANCE. Price **$2.00**

This book supplies, in a concise and available form, such facts and figures as are required by the Physician or Examiner to assist him in arriving at a correct estimate of the many contingencies upon which life insurance rests.

SWAIN (WILLIAM PAUL), F.R.C.S.,

Surgeon to the Royal Albert Hospital, Devonport.

SURGICAL EMERGENCIES: A MANUAL CONTAINING CONCISE DESCRIPTIONS OF VARIOUS ACCIDENTS AND EMERGENCIES, WITH DIRECTIONS FOR THEIR IMMEDIATE TREATMENT. With numerous Wood Engravings. In one volume, 12mo. Cloth. Price **$2.00**

STILLE (ALFRED), M. D.

Professor of the Theory and Practice of Medicine in the University of Pennsylvania, &c.

EPIDEMIC MENINGITIS; or, Cerebro-Spinal Meningitis.   In one volume, Octavo. $2.00

This monograph is a timely publication, comprehensive in its scope, and presenting within a small compass a fair digest of our existing knowledge of the disease, particularly acceptable at the present time.   It is just such a one as is needed, and may be taken as a model for similar works.— *American Journal Medical Sciences.*

SMITH (WILLIAM ROBERT),

Resident Surgeon, Hants County Hospital.

LECTURES ON THE EFFICIENT TRAINING OF NURSES FOR HOSPITAL AND PRIVATE WORK.   With Illustrations. 12mo.   Cloth.   Price $2.00

SMITH (HEYWOOD), M. D.,

Physician to the Hospital for Women, &c.

PRACTICAL GYNAECOLOGY.   A Hand-Book for Students and Practitioners.   With Illustrations.   Price $1.50

" It is obviously the work of a thoroughly intelligent practitioner, well versed in his art."
—*British Medical Journal.*

SANSOM (ARTHUR ERNEST), M.B.,

Physician to King's College Hospital, &c.

CHLOROFORM.   Its Action and Administration.   Price $1.50

BY SAME AUTHOR.

LECTURES ON THE PHYSICAL DIAGNOSIS OF DISEASES OF THE HEART, intended for Students and Practitioners. $1.50

SCANZONI (F. W. VON),

Professor in the University of Wurzburg.

A PRACTICAL TREATISE ON THE DISEASES OF THE SEXUAL ORGANS OF WOMEN.   Translated from the French. By A. K. GARDNER, M.D.   With Illustrations.   Octavo.   . $5.00

STOKES (WILLIAM),

Regius Professor of Physic in the University of Dublin.

THE DISEASES OF THE HEART AND THE AORTA. Octavo. $3.00

SYDENHAM SOCIETY'S PUBLICATIONS.   New Series, 1859 to 1878 inclusive, 20 years, 81 vols.   Subscriptions received, and back years furnished at $9.00 per year.   Full prospectus, with the Reports of the Society and a list of the Books published, furnished free upon application.

SANKEY (W. H. O.), M. D., F. R. C. P.

LECTURES ON MENTAL DISEASES.   Octavo .   . $3.00

SWERINGEN (HIRAM V.).
Member American Pharmaceutical Association, &c.

PHARMACEUTICAL LEXICON. A Dictionary of Pharmaceutical Science. Containing a concise explanation of the various subjects and terms of Pharmacy, with appropriate selections from the collateral sciences. Formulæ for officinal, empirical, and dietetic preparations; selections from the prescriptions of the most eminent physicians of Europe and America; an alphabetical list of diseases and their definitions; an account of the various modes in use for the preservation of dead bodies for interment or dissection; tables of signs and abbreviations, weights and measures, doses, antidotes to poisons, &c., &c. Designed as a guide for the Pharmaceutist, Druggist, Physician, &c. Royal Octavo.   Price in cloth $3.00
"   leather 4.00

SEWILL (H. E.), M. R. C. S., Eng., L. D. S.,
Dental Surgeon to the West London Hospital.

THE STUDENT'S GUIDE TO DENTAL ANATOMY AND SURGERY. With 77 Illustrations. Price $1.50

SHEPPARD (EDGAR), M. D.
Professor of Psychological Medicine in King's College, London.

MADNESS, IN ITS MEDICAL, SOCIAL, AND LEGAL ASPECTS. A series of Lectures delivered at King's College, London. Octavo. Price $2.25

SAVAGE (HENRY), M. D., F. R. C. S.
Consulting Physician to the Samaritan Free Hospital, London.

THE SURGERY, SURGICAL PATHOLOGY, and Surgical Anatomy of the Female Pelvic Organs, in a Series of Colored Plates taken from Nature: with Commentaries, Notes, and Cases. Third Edition, greatly enlarged. A quarto volume. Price . $12.00

SAVORY AND MOORE.

A CONDENSED COMPENDIUM OF DOMESTIC MEDICINE AND COMPANION TO THE MEDICINE CHEST. With Engravings. 12mo. Cloth. Price $0.50

SUTTON (FRANCIS), F. C. S.

A SYSTEMATIC HAND-BOOK OF VOLUMETRIC ANALYSIS, or the Quantitative Estimation of Chemical Substances by Measure, Applied to Liquids, Solids, and Gases. Third Edition, enlarged. With numerous Illustrations. Now Ready. Price .   . $5.00

SMITH (EUSTACE), M.D.
Physician to the East London Hospital for Diseases of Children, &c.

CLINICAL STUDIES OF DISEASES OF THE LUNGS IN CHILDREN. Price $2.50

TANNER (THOMAS HAWKES), M.D., F.R.C.P., &c.

THE PRACTICE OF MEDICINE. Sixth American from the last London Edition. Revised, much Enlarged, and thoroughly brought up to the present time. With a complete Section on the Diseases Peculiar to Women, an extensive Appendix of Formulæ for Medicines, Baths, &c., &c. Royal Octavo, over 1100 pages. Price, in cloth, $6.00; leather $7.00

There is a common character about the writings of Dr. Tanner—a characteristic which constitutes one of their chief values: they are all essentially and thoroughly practical. Dr. Tanner never, for one moment, allows this utilitarian end to escape his mental view. He aims at teaching how to recognize and how to cure disease, and in this he is thoroughly successful. . . . It is, indeed, a wonderful mine of knowledge. — *Medical Times.*

SAME AUTHOR.

A PRACTICAL TREATISE ON THE DISEASES OF INFANCY AND CHILDHOOD. Third American from the last London Edition, Revised and Enlarged. By ALFRED MEADOWS, M.D., London, M.R.C.P., Physician to the Hospital for Women and to the General Lying-in Hospital, &c., &c. Price $3.00

TANNER'S INDEX OF DISEASES AND THEIR TREATMENT. Second Edition. Carefully Revised. With many Additions and Improvements. By W. H. BROADBENT, M.D., F.R.C.P., Physician to the London Fever Hospital, &c., &c. Octavo. Cloth. $3.00

A MEMORANDA OF POISONS. A New and much Enlarged Edition. Price $0.75

TYSON (JAMES), M.D.,
Lecturer on Microscopy in the University of Pennsylvania, &c.

THE CELL DOCTRINE. Its History and Present State, with a Copious Bibliography of the Subject, for the use of Students of Medicine and Dentistry. With Colored Plate, and numerous Illustrations on Wood. Second Edition. Price $2.00

BY SAME AUTHOR.

A PRACTICAL GUIDE TO THE EXAMINATION OF URINE. For the use of Physicians and Students. With a Colored Plate and numerous Illustrations Engraved on Wood. Second Edition. Just Ready. Price $1.25

TAFT (JONATHAN), D.D.S.,
Professor of Operative Dentistry in the Ohio College, &c.

A PRACTICAL TREATISE ON OPERATIVE DENTISTRY. Third Edition, thoroughly Revised, with Additions, and fully brought up to the Present State of the Science. Containing over 100 Illustrations. Octavo. Price, in cloth, $4.25. In leather, . . $5.00

TURNBULL (LAURENCE), M.D.

THE ADVANTAGES AND ACCIDENTS OF ARTIFICIAL ANÆSTHESIA. A Manual of Anæsthetic Agents, Modes of Administration, etc. Second Edition, Enlarged. 25 Illustrations. Cloth. $1.50

THOMPSON (E. S.), M.D.,
Physician to Hospital for Consumption, etc.

COUGHS AND COLDS. Their Causes, Nature, and Treatment. 12mo. Cloth. Price $0.60

TROUSSEAU (A.),
Professor of Clinical Medicine to the Faculty of Medicine, Paris, &c.

LECTURES ON CLINICAL MEDICINE. Delivered at the Hôtel Dieu, Paris. Translated from the Third Revised and Enlarged Edition by P. VICTOR BAZIRE, M.D., London and Paris; and JOHN ROSE CORMACK, M.D., Edinburgh, F.R.S., &c. With a full Index, Table of Contents, &c. Complete in Two volumes, royal octavo, bound in cloth. Price $8.00; in Leather $10.00

Trousseau's Lectures have attained a reputation both in England and this country far greater than any work of a similar character heretofore written; and, notwithstanding but few medical men could afford to purchase the expensive edition issued by the Sydenham Society, it has had an extensive sale. In order, however, to bring the work within the reach of all the profession, the publishers now issue this edition, containing all the lectures as contained in the five-volume edition, at one-half the price. The *London Lancet*, in speaking of the work, says: "It treats of diseases of daily occurrence and of the most vital interest to the practitioner. And we should think any medical library absurdly incomplete now which did not have alongside of Watson, Graves, and Tanner, the 'Clinical Medicine' of Trousseau."

The Sydenham Society's Edition of Trousseau can also be furnished in sets, or in separate volumes, as follows: Volumes I., II., and III., $5.00 each. Volumes IV. and V., $4.00 each.

TILT (EDWARD JOHN), M.D.

THE CHANGE OF LIFE IN HEALTH AND DISEASE. A Practical Treatise on the Nervous and other Affections incidental to Women at the Decline of Life. Third London Edition. Price, $3.00

SAME AUTHOR.

A HAND-BOOK OF UTERINE THERAPEUTICS AND OF DISEASES OF WOMEN. Fourth London Edition. Price, $3.50

THOMPSON (SIR HENRY),
Emeritus Professor of Clinical Surgery, and Consulting Surgeon to University College Hospital.

CLINICAL LECTURES ON DISEASES OF THE URINARY ORGANS. Fifth Edition, Enlarged, with numerous additional Engravings. 8vo. $3.50

SAME AUTHOR.

ON THE PREVENTIVE TREATMENT OF CALCULOUS DISEASE, and the Use of Solvent Remedies. Second Edition. $1.00

PRACTICAL LITHOTOMY AND LITHOTRITY. Second Edition, with Illustrations. $3.50

THORNTON (W. PUGIN), M.D.
Surgeon to Hospital for Diseases of the Throat, &c.

ON TRACHEOTOMY, Especially in Relation to Diseases of the Larynx and Trachea. With Photographic and other Illustrations. Price $1.75

THOROWGOOD (JOHN C.), M.D.,
Lecturer on Materia Medica at the Middlesex Hospital.

THE STUDENT'S GUIDE TO MATERIA MEDICA. With Engravings on Wood. $2.00

TYLER SMITH (W.), M.D.,
Physician, Accoucheur, and Lecturer on Midwifery, &c.

ON OBSTETRICS. A Course of Lectures. Edited by A. K. GARDNER, M.D. With Illustrations. Octavo. . . . $5.00

THOROWGOOD (J. C.), M. D.,

Physician to the City of London Hospital for Diseases of the Chest, and to the West London Hospital, &c.

NOTES ON ASTHMA. Its various Forms, their Nature and Treatment, including Hay Asthma, with an Appendix of Formulæ, &c. Third Edition. Price $1.50

TIDY (C. MEYMOTT), M. D.,

Professor of Chemistry in London Hospital.

A HAND-BOOK OF MODERN CHEMISTRY, Organic and Inorganic. 8vo. 600 pages. Cloth, red edges. Price . . $5.00

TOMES (JOHN), F. R. S.

Late Dental Surgeon to the Middlesex and Dental Hospitals, &c.

A SYSTEM OF DENTAL SURGERY. The Second Revised and Enlarged Edition, by CHARLES S. TOMES, M.A., Lecturer on Dental Anatomy and Physiology, and Assistant Dental Surgeon to the Dental Hospital of London. With 263 Illustrations. Price . . $5.00

TOMES (C. S.), M. A.

Lecturer on Anatomy and Physiology, and Assistant Surgeon to the Dental Hospital of London.

A MANUAL OF DENTAL ANATOMY, HUMAN AND COMPARATIVE. With 179 Illustrations. Now Ready. Price . $3.50

TRANSACTIONS OF THE COLLEGE OF PHYSICIANS OF PHILADELPHIA. NEW SERIES.

VOLUMES I., II., III., & IV. Price, per volume . . . $2.50

THUDICHUM (JOHN L. W.), M. D.,

Lettsomian Professor of Medicine, Medical Society, London, &c.

ON PATHOLOGY OF THE URINE. Including a Complete Guide to Analysis. A new Revised and Enlarged Edition. With Illustrations. Octavo. Price $5.00

TOLAND (H. H.), M. D.,

Professor of the Principles and Practice of Surgery in the University of California.

LECTURES ON PRACTICAL SURGERY. Second Edition. With Additions and numerous Illustrations. Price, in cloth, $4.50
" in leather, 5.00

TIBBITS (HERBERT), M. D.

Medical Superintendent of the National Hospital for the Paralyzed and Epileptic, &c.

A HANDBOOK OF MEDICAL ELECTRICITY. With Sixty-four large Illustrations. Small octavo. Price . . . $1.50

The author of this volume is the translator of Duchenne's great work on "Localized Electrization." Avoiding contested points in electro-physiology and therapeutics, he has prepared this handbook as containing all that is essential for the busy practitioner to know, not only when, but in EXPLICIT AND FULL DETAIL, how to use Electricity in the treatment of disease, and to make the practitioner as much at home in the use of his electrical as his other medical instruments.

VIRCHOW (RUDOLI·HE), Professor, University of Berlin.

CELLULAR PATHOLOGY. 144 Illustrations. Octavo. $5.00

BY SAME AUTHOR.

POST-MORTEM EXAMINATIONS. A Description and Explanation of the Method of Performing Them in the Dead House of the Berlin Charité Hospital. Price $0.75

ARTHUR VACHER, Translator and Editor of Fresenius's Chemical Analysis.

A PRIMER OF CHEMISTRY. Including Analysis. 18mo. Cloth. Price $0.50

WARING (EDWARD JOHN), F.R.C.S., F.L.S., &c., &c.

PRACTICAL THERAPEUTICS. Considered chiefly with reference to Articles of the Materia Medica. Third American from the last London Edition. Price, in cloth, $4.00; leather . . $5.00

There are many features in Dr. Waring's Therapeutics which render it especially valuable to the Practitioner and Student of Medicine, much important and reliable information being found in it not contained in similar works; also in its completeness, the convenience of its arrangement, and the greater prominence given to the medicinal application of the various articles of the Materia Medica in the treatment of morbid conditions of the Human Body, &c. It is divided into two parts, the alphabetical arrangement being adopted throughout. It contains also an excellent INDEX OF DISEASES, with a list of the medicines applicable as remedies, and a full INDEX of the medicines and preparations noticed in the work.

WYTHE (JOSEPH H), A.M., M.D., &c.

THE PHYSICIAN'S POCKET, DOSE, AND SYMPTOM BOOK. Containing the Doses and Uses of all the PrincipalArticles of the Materia Medica, and Original Preparations; A Table of Weights and Measures, Rules to Proportion the Doses of Medicines, Common Abbreviations used in Writing Prescriptions, Table of Poisons and Antidotes, Classification of the Materia Medica, Dietetic Preparations, Table of Symptomatology, Outlines of General Pathology and Therapeutics, &c. The Eleventh Revised Edition. Price, in cloth, $1.00; in leather, tucks, with pockets, ... $1.25

BY SAME AUTHOR.

THE MICROSCOPIST, a Compendium of Microscopic Science, Micro-Mineralogy, Micro-Chemistry, Biology, Histology, and Pathological Histology. Elegantly Illustrated. Price . . . $4.00

WILKS AND MOXON.

LECTURES ON PATHOLOGICAL ANATOMY. By SAMUEL WILKS, M.D., F.R.S., Physician to, and Lecturer on Medicine at, Guy's Hospital. Second Edition, Enlarged and Revised. By WALTER MOXON, M.D., F.R.S., Physician to, and late Lecturer on Pathology at, Guy's Hospital. $6.00

WILSON (ERASMUS), F.R.S.

HEALTHY SKIN. A Popular Treatise on the Skin and Hair, their Preservation and Management. Eighth Edition. Cloth. . $1.00

WILSON (GEORGE), M. A., M. D.

Medical Officer to the Convict Prison at Portsmouth.

A HANDBOOK OF HYGIENE AND SANITARY SCIENCE.
With Engravings. Third Edition, carefully Revised. Containing Chapters on Public Health, Food, Air, Ventilation and Warming, Water, Water Analysis, Dwellings, Hospitals, Removal, Purification, Utilization of Sewage and Effects on Public Health, Drainage, Epidemics, Duties of Medical Officers of Health, &c., &c. Price $3.00

WAGSTAFFE (WILLIAM WARWICK), F. R. C. S.

Assistant-Surgeon and Lecturer on Anatomy at St. Thomas's Hospital.

THE STUDENT'S GUIDE TO HUMAN OSTEOLOGY. With Twenty-three Lithographic Plates and Sixty Wood Engravings. 12mo. Cloth. Price $3.00

WARD ON AFFECTIONS OF THE LIVER AND INTESTINAL CANAL; with Remarks on Ague, Scurvy, Purpura, &c. $2.00

WHEELER (C. GILBERT), M. D.,

Professor of Chemistry in the University of Chicago.

MEDICAL CHEMISTRY: Including the Outlines of Organic and Physiological Chemistry. Based in Part upon Riche's Manual De Chimie. Octavo. Cloth. Price $3.00

WILSON (JOSEPH C.), M. D.,

Physician to the Philadelphia Hospital, &c.

THE SUMMER AND ITS DISEASES. (Vol. III., American Health Primers.) Cloth. Price $0.50

WOAKES (EDWARD), M. D.

ON DEAFNESS, GIDDINESS, AND NOISES IN THE HEAD.
With Illustrations. Price $1.25

WEDL (CARL), M. D.,

Professor of Histology, &c., in the University of Vienna.

DENTAL PATHOLOGY. The Pathology of the Teeth. With Special Reference to their Anatomy and Physiology. With Notes by Thos. B. Hitchcock, M.D., Prof. of Dental Pathology, Harvard University, Cambridge. 105 Illustrations. Cloth, $3.50; Leather, $4.50

WEST (CHARLES), M. D., F. R. C. P.

LECTURES ON THE DISEASES OF WOMEN. Revised and in part Rewritten by the Author. With numerous Additions by J. Matthews Duncan, M. D., Obstetric Physician to St. Bartholomew's Hospital. Fourth London Edition. Octavo. Price . . $5.00

WILKES (SAMUEL), M. D.,

Physician to, and Lecturer at, Guy's Hospital.

LECTURES ON DISEASES OF THE NERVOUS SYSTEM.
Delivered at Guy's Hospital. With Additions. Numerous Illustrative Cases, etc. $5.00

WOODMAN and TIDY.

A TEXT-BOOK OF FORENSIC MEDICINE AND TOXI-
COLOGY. By W. Bathurst Woodman, M. D., St. And., Assistant
Physician and Lecturer on Physiology at the London Hospital ; and C.
Meymott Tidy, M. A., M. B., Lecturer on Chemistry, and Professor
of Medical Jurisprudence and Public Health, at the London Hospital.
With Numerous Illustrations. Now ready, cloth, $7.50 ; leather, $8.50

WELLS (J. SŒLBERG), *Author's Edition*,
Ophthalmic Surgeon to King's College Hospital, &c.

TREATISE ON THE DISEASES OF THE EYE. Illustrated by
Ophthalmoscopic Plates and numerous Engravings on Wood. The
Fourth London Edition. Cloth,   Leather .   .   .

This is the author's own edition, printed in London under his supervision, and issued in
this country by special arrangement with him.

SAME AUTHOR.

ON LONG, SHORT, AND WEAK SIGHT, and their Treatment
by the Scientific Use of Spectacles. Fourth Edition Revised, with
Additions and numerous Illustrations. Price   .   .   . $2.25

WRIGHT (HENRY G.), M. D.,
Member of the Royal College of Physicians, &c.

ON HEADACHES. Their Causes and their Cure. From the London Edition. Seventh Thousand $0 50

WILSON (JOSEPH), M. D.,
Medical Director, U. S. N.

NAVAL HYGIENE — Human Health and the Means of Preventing Disease. With Illustrative Incidents derived from Naval Experience. Second Edition. With Colored Lithographs and other Illustrations. Octavo. Price $3.00

WALTON (HAYNES),
Surgeon In Charge of the Ophthalmic Department of, and Lecturer on Ophthalmic Medicine and Surgery
in, St. Mary's Hospital.

A PRACTICAL TREATISE ON DISEASES OF THE EYE,
Third Edition. Rewritten and enlarged. With five plain, and three
colored full-page plates, numerous Illustrations on Wood, Test Types,
&c., &c. Octavo volume of nearly 1200 pages. Price   . $9.00

WATERS (A. T. H.), M.D., F.R.C.P., &c.

DISEASES OF THE CHEST. Contributions to their Clinical History, Pathology, and Treatment. Second Edition, Revised and Enlarged.
With numerous Illustrative Cases and Chapters on Hæmoptysis, Hay
Fever, Thoracic Aneurism, and the Use of Chloral in certain Diseases
of the Chest, and Plates. Octavo. Price $4.00

WALKER (ALEXANDER),
Author of "Woman," "Beauty," &c.

INTERMARRIAGE; or, the Mode in which, and the Causes why,
Beauty, Health, Intellect result from certain Unions, and Deformity,
Disease, and Insanity from others. With Illustrations. 12mo. $1.00

AMERICAN HEALTH PRIMERS.

Edited by W. W. KEEN, M.D.,

Fellow of the College Physicians, Philadelphia, Surgeon to St. Mary's Hospital, &c.

It is one of the chief merits of the Medical Profession in modern times that its members are in the fore-front of every movement to prevent disease. It is due to them that the Science of what has been happily called " Preventive Medicine" has its existence. Not only in large cities, but in every town and hamlet, the Doctor leads in every effort to eradicate the sources of disease. These efforts have been ably seconded by intelligent and public-spirited citizens of many callings. The American Public Health Association and the Social Science Association, with their manifold and most useful influences, are organizations which have sprung from, and still further extend and reinforce, the efforts to improve the public health.

But the great mass of the public scarcely recognize the importance of such efforts, or, if they do, are ignorant of the facts of Anatomy, Physiology, and Hygiene, and of their practical application to the betterment of their health and the prevention of disease. Such knowledge does not come by nature. In most cases, in fact, it is a direct result of the most laborious research and the highest skill. Accordingly, it is the object of this series of American Health Primers to diffuse as widely and as cheaply as possible, among all classes, a knowledge of the elementary facts of Preventive Medicine, and the bearings and applications of the latest and best researches in every branch of Medical and Hygienic Science. They are not intended (save incidentally) to assist in curing disease, but to teach people how to take care of themselves, their children, their pupils, and their employès.

The series is written from the American standpoint, and with especial reference to our Climate, Architecture, Legislation, and modes of Life; and in all these respects we differ materially from other nations. Sanitary Legislation especially, which in England has made such notable progress, has barely begun with us, and it is hoped that the American Health Primers may assist in developing a public sentiment favorable to proper sanitary laws, especially in our large cities.

The subjects selected are of vital and practical importance in every-day life. They are treated in as popular a style as is consistent with their nature, technical terms being avoided as far as practicable. Each volume, if the subject calls for it, will be fully illustrated, so that the text may be clearly and readily understood by any one heretofore entirely ignorant of the structure and functions of the body. The authors have been selected with great care, and on account of special fitness, each for his subject, by reason of its previous careful study, either privately or as public teachers.

Dr. W. W. Keen has undertaken the supervision of the series as Editor, but it will be understood that he is not responsible for the statements or opinions of the individual authors.

SIX VOLUMES are NOW READY, others are in Press.

I. Hearing, and How to Keep It.	By CHAS. H. BURNETT, M.D., of Philada., *Surgeon in charge of Phila. Disp. for Diseases of the Ear. Aurist to Presbyterian Hospital, etc.*
II. Long Life, and How to Reach It.	By J. G. RICHARDSON, M.D., of Philada., *Prof. of Hygiene in University of Penna., etc.*
III. Sea Air and Sea Bathing.	By JOHN H. PACKARD, M.D., of Philada., *Surgeon to the Episcopal Hospital, etc.*
IV. The Summer and its Diseases.	By JAMES C. WILSON, M.D., of Philada., *Lecturer on Physical Diagnosis in Jefferson Medical College, etc.*
V. Eyesight, and How to Care for It.	By GEORGE C. HARLAN, M.D., of Phila., *Surgeon to the Wills (Eye) Hospital.*
VI. The Throat and the Voice.	By J. SOLIS COHEN, M.D., of Philada., *Lecturer on Diseases of the Throat in Jefferson Medical College.*
VII. The Winter and its Dangers.	By HAMILTON OSGOOD, M.D., of Boston, *Editorial Staff Boston Med. and Surg. Journal.*
VIII. The Mouth and the Teeth.	By J. W. WHITE, M.D., D.D.S., of Philada., *Editor of the Dental Cosmos.*
IX. Our Homes.	By HENRY HARTSHORNE, M.D., of Phila., *Formerly Prof. of Hygiene in Univer. of Penna.*
X. The Skin in Health and Disease.	By L. D. BULKLEY, M.D., of New York., *Physician to the Skin Department of the Dewitt Dispensary and of the New York Hospital.*
XI. Brain Work and Overwork.	By H. C. WOOD, Jr., M.D., of Philada., *Clinical Professor of Nervous Diseases in the University of Pennsylvania, etc.*

Other volumes are in preparation, including the following subjects: **"Preventable Diseases," " Accidents and Emergencies," "The Towns we Live In," "Diet in Health and Disease," "The Art of Nursing," "School and Industrial Hygiene,"** etc., etc. They will be 16mo in size, neatly printed on tinted paper, and handsomely bound in embossed cloth. Price, 50 cents.

Mailed free upon receipt of price.

Published by PRESLEY BLAKISTON, Philadelphia.

Milton Keynes UK
Ingram Content Group UK Ltd.
UKHW040926180224
437992UK00003B/67